DEJA REVIEW™
Physiology

NOTICE

DEJA REVIEW™
Physiology

Second Edition

Edward R. Gould, MD

Resident Physician
Department of Internal Medicine
Vanderbilt University
Nashville, Tennessee

SUNY Upstate Medical University
Syracuse, New York
Class of 2009

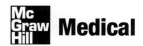 Medical

New York   Chicago   San Francisco   Lisbon   London   Madrid   Mexico City
Milan   New Delhi   San Juan   Seoul   Singapore   Sydney   Toronto

Déjà Review™: Physiology, Second Edition

1 2 3 4 5 6 7 8 9 0   DOC/DOC   14 13 12 11 10

ISBN 978-0-07-162725-2
MHID 0-07-162725-1

This book was set in Palatino by Glyph International.

The editors were Kirsten Funk and Peter J. Boyle.

The production supervisor was Catherine H. Saggese.

Project management was provided by Shruti Vasishta, Glyph International.

RR Donnelley was printer and binder.

This book is printed on acid-free paper.

Library of Congress Cataloging-in-Publication Data

Gould, Edward R.
      Deja review. Physiology / Edward R. Gould.—2nd ed.
          p. ; cm.—(Deja review)
      Rev. ed. of: Deja review. Physiology / David W. Lin ... [et al.]. c2006.
      Includes bibliographical references and index.
      ISBN-13: 978-0-07-162725-2 (pbk. : alk. paper)
      ISBN-10: 0-07-162725-1 (pbk. : alk. paper)   1. Human physiology—Examinations, questions, etc.   2. Physicians—Licenses—United States—Examinations—Study guides.
  I. Deja review. Physiology.   II. Title.   III. Title: Physiology.   IV. Series: Deja review.
      [DNLM: 1. Physiological Phenomena—Examination Questions.   QT 18.2
  G694d   2010]
      QP40.D45 2010
      612.0076—dc22
                                                                          2010006321

I would like to thank my family, always there with words of support or good food, whichever I needed more. A special thanks to my grandmother for instilling in me an intellectual hunger that has driven me through many a long night. It is our most important job to teach those who will follow us. I hope that this text is one small step toward that end.
—Edward R. Gould, MD

I would like to thank my mom, sister, and grandma who taught me the importance of perspective and perseverance. To Mary Lou and Rob whose unconditional support made the journey possible. And to my father, whose kind and compassionate heart will never be forgotten.
—Amy L. O'Brian, MD

To my friends, family and Hill. Thanks for all the help along the way!
—Joseph Resti, MD

Contents

Contributing Authors

Amy L. O'Brian, MD
Resident Pediatrician
Department of Pediatrics
University of Wisconsin
Madison, Wisconsin

SUNY Upstate Medical University
Syracuse, New York
Class of 2009

Joseph Resti, MD
Resident Anesthesiologist
Department of Anesthesia
University of Pittsburgh
Pittsburgh, Pennsylvania

SUNY Upstate Medical University
Syracuse, New York
Class of 2009

Faculty Reviewers

Steven Grassl, PhD
Department of Pharmacology
SUNY Upstate Medical University
Syracuse, New York

Student Reviewers

Max Gallegos
University of Kansas School of Medicine
Class of 2011

Sheree Perron
Eastern Virginia Medical School
Class of 2010

Preface

The main objective of a medical student preparing for Step 1 of the United States Medical Licensing Examination (USMLE) is to commit a vast body of knowledge to memory. Having recently prepared for Step 1, we realize how daunting this task can be. We feel there are two main guidelines that will allow you to be successful in your preparation for Step 1: (1) repetition of key facts and (2) using review questions to gauge your comprehension and memory. The Déjà Review™ series is a unique resource that has been designed to allow you to review the essential facts and determine your level of knowledge of the different subjects tested in Step 1. We also know, from experience, that building a solid foundation in the basic sciences (like with this physiology review book) will allow you to make a smooth transition into the clinical years of medical school.

ORGANIZATION

All concepts are presented in a question and answer format that covers the key facts on hundreds of commonly tested physiology topics that may appear on the USMLE Step 1 exam. The material is divided into chapters organized by physiologic systems along with a special chapter at the end that incorporates the material with its clinical presentation and relevance. Special emphasis has been placed on the pathways that govern the physiologic processes, as these areas are vital for comprehension of how the various systems work and how they can go awry, and they are the basis for the majority of questions in both your medical school course and Step 1.

The question and answer format has several important advantages:

- It provides a rapid, straightforward way for you to assess your strengths and weaknesses.
- It serves as a quick, last-minute review of high-yield facts.
- It allows you to efficiently review and commit to memory a large body of information.

At the end of each chapter, you will find clinical vignettes that expose you to the prototypic presentation of diseases classically tested on the USMLE Step 1. These board-style questions put the basic science into a clinical context, allowing you to apply the facts you have just reviewed in a clinical scenario and "Make the Diagnosis."

HOW TO USE THIS BOOK

This text was assembled with the intention of representing the core topics tested on course examinations and USMLE Step 1. Remember, this text is not intended to replace comprehensive textbooks, course packs, or lectures. It is simply intended to serve as a supplement to your studies during your physiology course work and Step 1 preparation. You may use the book to quiz yourself or classmates on topics covered in recent lectures and clinical case discussions. A bookmark is included so that you can easily cover up the answers as you work through each chapter. The compact, condensed design of the book is conducive to studying on the go, especially during any downtime throughout your day.

We encourage you to begin using this book early in your first year to reinforce topics covered on your course examinations.

However you choose to study, we hope you find this resource helpful throughout your preclinical years and during your preparation for USLME Step 1. Best of luck!

Ed, Amy, and Joe

Acknowledgments

It is my pleasure to recognize the faculty and staff of Upstate Medical University for their outstanding teaching and their interest in—and dedication to—the education of their students.

A special thanks to Dr. Steven Grassl from the Department of Pharmacology at Upstate Medical University for his tireless effort toward improving the content of this book. While our visits were usually about this text with discussion aimed at topical clarity and content improvement, they always included refreshing conversation; he has my personal thanks for both.

Finally, the contributing authors and I would also like to thank our editor, Kirsten Funk, for her patience, kindness, and guidance through this process.

Edward R. Gould

CHAPTER 1

General Physiology

CELL MEMBRANES AND TRANSPORT ACROSS MEMBRANES

What are the components of a cell membrane?

1. Cholesterol
2. Phospholipids
3. Sphingolipids
4. Glycolipids
5. Proteins

Which cell membrane component contributes the most to stability?

Cholesterol

What are the two molecular components of cell membrane phospholipids?

Glycerol backbone (hydrophilic) and fatty acid chains (hydrophobic)

How are integral and peripheral proteins different?

Integral: span entire membrane

Peripheral: located on either side of the membrane

How are integral proteins attached to the membrane?

Hydrophobic interactions with the phospholipid bilayer

Give some examples of integral and peripheral proteins:

Integral: ion channels, transport proteins

Peripheral: spectrin, ferrochelatase (an example of a membrane-linked enzyme)

How do lipid-soluble substances move across cell membranes?

Simple diffusion across the hydrophobic lipid bilayer

How do water-soluble substances move across cell membranes?

Cross through water-filled channels or transported by carriers, as they cannot dissolve in the lipid bilayer

What are the different types of transport across a cell membrane?

Simple diffusion, facilitated diffusion, primary active transport, and secondary active transport

Which types of cellular transport are carrier mediated?

Facilitated diffusion, primary active transport, and secondary active transport

Which types of cellular transport require metabolic energy?

Primary active transport and secondary active transport

What is an example of a primary active transporter?

Any ion-translocating ATPase

What are the two subtypes of secondary active transporters?

1. Cotransport
2. Countertransport

What is cotransport (symport)?

Mediated transfer of two or more solutes in the same direction across a cell membrane

What is countertransport (antiport)?

Mediated transfer of two or more solutes in opposite directions across a cell membrane

Explain secondary active transport:

It couples the transfer of two or more solutes across a membrane; one solute moves down its electrochemical gradient providing the motive force for movement of the other solute(s) against its electrochemical gradient

Which ion most often functions as the motive force for secondary active transport?

Na^+; it has a favorable inward gradient across almost all cell membranes

What is the direction of solute movement relative to the electrochemical gradient in the following types of transport?

Simple diffusion

Downhill

Facilitated diffusion

Downhill

Primary active transport

Uphill

Secondary active: cotransport and countertransport

For both types of transport one solute moves down its gradient providing energy for the other solutes to move against their gradients. In cotransport, solutes move in the same direction. In countertransport, they move in opposite directions.

What does permeability describe?	Ease with which a solute is able to diffuse across a membrane
What factors can increase membrane permeability?	1. Increased oil/water partition coefficient 2. Decreased size of solute 3. Decreased membrane thickness
What are the characteristics that are important in carrier-mediated transport?	Stereospecificity, saturation, and inhibition (competitive, noncompetitive)
What is the transport rate when the carriers are saturated?	Transport maximum (T_m)
Which is faster, diffusion or facilitated diffusion of a hydrophilic solute?	Facilitated diffusion, as it is carrier mediated
Which has unlimited (theoretically) capacity for cellular transport?	Diffusion, it is limited only by its gradient and its permeability characteristics

Na$^+$-K$^+$ PUMP

What is the Na$^+$-K$^+$ pump?	An integral membrane protein mediating ATP hydrolysis as energy for Na$^+$-K$^+$ exchange
What does the Na$^+$-K$^+$ pump *do*?	Extrudes 3 Na$^+$ from within the cell and takes in 2 K$^+$ from outside the cell
Is the Na$^+$-K$^+$ pump electroneutral?	No; the Na$^+$-K$^+$ pump is electrogenic, mediating net efflux of positive charge creating a negatively charged interior of the cell.
What provides the energy for the Na$^+$-K$^+$ pump?	Hydrolysis of adenosine triphosphate (ATP)
What example substances inhibit activity of the Na$^+$-K$^+$ ATPase pump?	Ouabain and digitalis glycosides

INTERCELLULAR CONNECTIONS

What are some examples of intercellular connections?	Tight junctions, gap junctions, and desmosomes

What is the role of tight junctions? (Histology often calls these zonula occludens.)	Circumferential bands of proteins that impede the movement of solute paracellularly
Tight junctions have been classically divided into tight and leaky epithelia. Explain the difference and give examples:	Tight: many bands of protein blocking all (most) paracellular movement of water and solute; found in the ascending limb of the loop of Henle
	Leaky: few bands of protein, allows paracellular movement of water; found in the proximal tubule and throughout the gut
What is the role of desmosomes? (Histology often calls these zonula adherens.)	These are regions of connections between adjacent cells. They permit paracellular movement, but do not allow for cell-to-cell flow.
What is the role of gap junctions?	Protein bridges from one cell to an adjacent cell. These allow for solute flow between adjacent cells.
What important tissue relies on gap junctions for proper function?	Myocardium, allow for rapid conduction of electrical impulses

OSMOSIS

Define osmolarity:	Concentration of osmotically active particles in a solution
Define osmosis:	Flow of water across a semipermeable membrane from a low osmolarity compartment to a compartment with a higher osmolarity
Define osmotic pressure:	The hydrostatic pressure necessary to counter osmosis between two compartments
How is osmotic pressure calculated?	Van't Hoff's law: $$\pi = gCRT$$ π = osmotic pressure (mm Hg), g = number of particles in solution (osm/mol), C = concentration (mol/L), R = gas constant (0.082 L · atm/mol · K), T = absolute temperature (K)

What is oncotic pressure?	Osmotic pressure created by proteins (e.g., colloid osmotic pressure)
What is tonicity?	The relative difference in osmolarity in different compartments
What are hypotonic and hypertonic solutions?	These terms refer to the relationship between two compartments. Hypotonicity refers to a relatively lower osmolarity of one compartment to another. Hypertonicity, likewise, refers to a solution having higher osmolarity than another.
How does infusion of hypo/hypertonic solutions influence fluid compartments?	Infusion of a hypotonic solution into the intravascular space will initially decrease osmolarity, and water will tend to move into the interstitium, increasing edema. Infusion of hypertonic fluids will lead to the opposite effect.

MEMBRANE POTENTIALS

Define steady state:	The stable condition between biologic compartments when the *net* ionic flow is zero
Define diffusion potential:	Potential difference across a membrane due to the separation of positive and negative charge across a membrane
What determines the size of the diffusion potential?	The magnitude of the ionic charge separation
Can a diffusion potential be generated if the membrane is not permeable to the ion?	No
What determines the sign of the diffusion potential?	The direction of the positive and negative charge separation across the membrane
True or False? Creation of the diffusion potential requires the movement of a significant number of ions.	False. The separation of very few ions creates a diffusion potential.
What facilitates the movement of ions across the membrane?	Typically, ion channels, but also pumps and carrier transporters

What controls the opening and closing of ion channels?

A molecular gating mechanism

What are the three general components of an ion channel?

1. The pore
2. The selectivity filter
3. The gating mechanism

What is the selectivity filter?

Grants specificity to the various channels, allowing only one type of ion through the channel

What does the conductance of an ion channel depend on?

The probability that the channel is open and its capacity to mediate translocation through the pore

What types of ion channel gating mechanisms are there?

Voltage-sensitive, ligand-induced, and mechanical gates.

What controls the opening of voltage-gated channels?

Membrane potential

What controls the opening and closing of ligand-gated channels?

Hormones

Second messengers

Neurotransmitters

What controls the opening of mechanical gates?

Membrane stretch and manipulation. Commonly seen in epithelial layers.

Define equilibrium potential (*E*):

Electrical potential that exactly opposes diffusion caused by an ionic concentration difference. (In other words: how much energy do we have to use to *stop* diffusion)

What is it called when the electrical and chemical driving forces of an ion are equally opposed?

Electrochemical equilibrium

What equation is used to calculate equilibrium potentials?

Nernst equation:

$$E = -2.3 \frac{RT}{zF} \log_{10} \frac{[C_i]}{C_e}$$

E = equilibrium potential (mV),
2.3 RT/F = constants (60 mV at 37°C)
z = charge on the ion
C_i = intracellular concentration (mM)
C_e = extracellular concentration (mM)

What are the approximate values of the equilibrium potential for the following ions in nerves and muscles?

Na^+	+65 mV
K^+	−85 mV
Ca^{2+}	+120 mV
Cl^-	−85 mV

Define the resting membrane potential.
Electrical potential across a semipermeable membrane when the cell is at steady state

Is energy consumed to generate the resting membrane potential?
Yes, the maintenance of the ionic gradients requires constant energy input

Define depolarization:
Membrane potential becomes less negative (i.e., −60 mV → −40 mV)

Define hyperpolarization:
Membrane potential becomes more negative (i.e., −60 mV → −90 mV)

What is a cell called if it is capable of producing an action potential?
Excitable

What do action potentials consist of?
Rapid depolarization and repolarization

What are the unique characteristics of action potentials?
All-or-none events, propagation, and stereotypical size and shape (differs for different cells, e.g., cardiac versus neurons but always reproducible in each cell type)

What is the point after which an action potential is inevitable?
Threshold

What does inward or outward current charge refer to?
Movement of positive charge into (inward) and out of (outward) the cell

What is the resting membrane potential for nerve cells?
−70 mV

What ion is primarily responsible for the resting membrane potential of nerve cells?
K^+

Why does K^+ contribute the most to the resting potential?
At rest, K^+ has the greatest ionic conductance

What signals the activation gates of Na⁺ channels?	Depolarization of the cell membrane; these are voltage-gated channels
What ion is responsible for the upstroke of the action potential in nerve cells?	Na⁺
Define overshoot:	Peak of the action potential at which the membrane potential is positive
What signals the inactivation gates of Na⁺ channels?	Depolarization of the cell membrane
How can depolarization cause both activation and deactivation of Na⁺ channel gates?	Inactivation occurs more slowly than activation
What causes repolarization of the cell membrane following an action potential?	As the inward Na⁺ conductance falls due to channel inactivation, outward K⁺ conductance leads to repolarization
What signals the opening of K⁺ channels during an action potential?	Depolarization of the cell membrane
What is the hyperpolarization of the afterpotential called?	Undershoot
What causes undershoot?	K⁺ channels stay open after the Na⁺ channels close

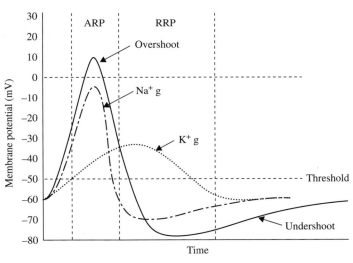

Figure 1.1 Action potential: ionic conductance.

What types of refractory periods are there?	Absolute and relative
In what type of refractory period can an action potential not be elicited?	Absolute refractory period
With what does the duration of the absolute refractory period coincide?	The duration of action potential (AP) propagation
What produces the absolute refractory period?	The inactivated Na^+ channels cannot participate in a new action potential
How can an action potential be elicited during the relative refractory period?	With a larger than usual stimulus to produce a larger inward current. Remember, the Na^+ channels are now competing with the K^+ channels.
What is the duration of the relative refractory period?	Starts at the end of the absolute refractory period and lasts until the cell returns to its resting potential
How do action potentials propagate?	By spread of local currents to adjacent areas of the membrane
What ensures that an action potential will propagate only in the forward direction?	The areas that it has already moved through are refractory and cannot support new action potentials
How can conduction velocity be increased?	Increased fiber diameter and myelination
What type of conduction do myelinated axons demonstrate?	Saltatory
What type of a substance is myelin, insulating or conductive?	Insulating
Where are action potentials maintained in myelinated axons?	Nodes of Ranvier
Describe salutatory conduction:	A depolarizing current rapidly moves from node to node because the insulating myelin does not allow ionic flow.

Which has faster conduction, myelinated or unmyelinated fibers?

Myelinated fibers (conduction is up to 50 times faster)

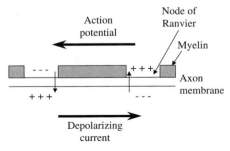

Figure 1.2 Saltatory conduction.

SYNAPTIC TRANSMISSION

As action potentials arrive at the presynaptic terminal they lead to depolarization. What does that depolarization stimulate in the presynaptic cell?

The release of neurotransmitter

The influx of this ion into the presynaptic terminal is directly responsible for presynaptic vesicle release.

Ca^+; it enters through voltage-gated Ca^+ channels that are triggered by the arrival of the action potential

The space that neurotransmitter is released into is called what?

Synaptic cleft

What do neurotransmitters bind to?

Receptors on the cell membrane of the postsynaptic (most common) and/or presynaptic cell

What action do neurotransmitters have on postsynaptic cells?

Binding to their receptor causes a *receptor-specific* change in the membrane's ionic permeability and thereby the membrane potential

What effect do they have on the presynaptic terminal?

Modulation of the synaptic transmission. Can facilitate or inhibit continued neurotransmitter release

Describe the numbered processes in Figure 1.3:

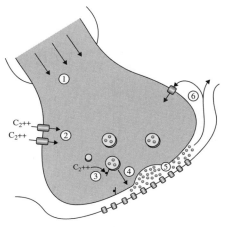

1. Arrival of action potential
2. Opening of voltage-gated Ca^{++} channels followed by Ca^{++}
3. Ca^{++} binds to synaptotagmin to initiate vesicle fusion
4. Exocytosis of vesicle contents
5. Extruded neurotransmitter binds to postsynaptic cell
6. Synapse is cleared of neurotransmitter by reuptake, or hydrolysis

Figure 1.3 Synaptic transmission.

If a neurotransmitter is *inhibitory*, what does it do to the postsynaptic cell?

Hyperpolarize postsynaptic membrane

If a neurotransmitter is *excitatory*, what does it do to the postsynaptic cell?

Depolarize postsynaptic membrane

What is it called when the many miniature end-plate potentials combine to produce the final end-plate potential?

Summation; this is the process of *integration* of many stimuli

What types of summation are there?

Spatial summation and temporal summation

Define spatial summation:

Two excitatory inputs from *different inputs* arrive *simultaneously* at the postsynaptic terminal and produce a greater depolarization

Define temporal summation:

Two excitatory inputs from the *same input* arrive *back-to-back* at the postsynaptic terminal and produce a stepwise increase in depolarization due to their overlap

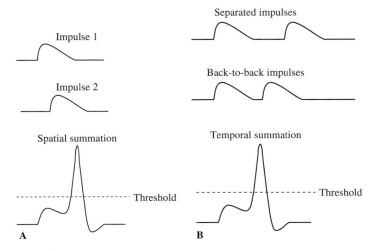

Figure 1.4   Summation. A. Spatial summation. B. Temporal summation.

What is it called when there is a single presynaptic element for each postsynaptic element?

One-to-one synapse

What is it called when there are many presynaptic elements for each postsynaptic element?

Many-to-one synapse

What happens when a many-to-one synapse receives both excitatory and inhibitory signals?

The postsynaptic cell integrates all of the signals and may or may not fire an action potential (AP)

What must be reached for the postsynaptic cell to fire an AP?

Threshold

What are the excitatory and inhibitory signals called in a many-to-one synapse?

Excitatory postsynaptic potential (EPSP) and inhibitory postsynaptic potential (IPSP)

What does an EPSP cause?

Opening of Na$^+$ channels, which leads to depolarization

What does an IPSP cause?

Opening of either K$^+$ or Cl$^-$ channels, which leads to hyperpolarization

Why is Na$^+$ movement depolarizing, but K$^+$ movement is hyperpolarizing when they're both positively charged?

The ions will move down their gradients. Na$^+$ moves in, K$^+$ moves out.

What neurotransmitters are classically considered excitatory?

Acetylcholine (Ach), norepinephrine (NE), epinephrine (Epi), dopamine (DA), glutamate (Glu), and serotonin (5-HT)

What neurotransmitters are classically considered inhibitory?

γ-Aminobutyric acid (GABA) and glycine

Neurotransmitters

What determines if a neurotransmitter is excitatory or inhibitory?

The receptor!

Which excitatory neurotransmitter is most prevalent in the brain?

Glutamate

What types of receptors does glutamate bind to?

Kainite receptor, NMDA receptor, and AMPA receptor

What ions can move through glutamate receptors?

Na$^+$, Ca^{++}, and K$^+$ ion channels

Which type of above receptor produces a longer, slower ionic current?

NMDA; this is the channel type that allows Ca^{++} in addition to the monovalent cations

If extracellular glutamate concentration rises, what can happen?

Neuronal excitotoxicity

What is GABA synthesized from?

Glutamate

What catalyzes GABA synthesis?

Glutamate decarboxylase

What occurs when GABA binds to the following receptors?

GABA$_A$ receptor

Increases Cl$^-$ conductance

GABA$_B$ receptor

Increases K$^+$ conductance; G-protein coupled

Which GABA receptor is the site of action for barbiturates and benzodiazepines?

$GABA_A$ receptor

Where is glycine primarily found?

Spinal cord and brain stem

What effect does glycine cause when it binds to its receptor?

Increases Cl^- conductance

Dopamine, norepinephrine, epinephrine (all catecholamines) as well as histamine and serotonin are all considered part of what class of molecules?

Biogenic amines

How are biogenic amine neurotransmitters cleared from the synaptic cleft?

Reuptake into both presynaptic terminal and adjacent glia by specific transporters

How are they degraded after reuptake?

Monoamine oxidase, as well as catechol-O-methyl transferase

Diagram the synthetic pathway for dopamine, NE, and Epi. (focus on the products and let the enzymes fall into place)

Tyrosine
↓ *tyrosine hydroxylase*
L-Dopa
↓ *dopa decarboxylase*
Dopamine
↓ *dopamine β-hydroxylase*
Norepinephrine
↓ *phenylethanolamine-N-methyltransferase*
Epinephrine

What type of fiber releases NE?

Postganglionic sympathetic fibers; the exception being those fibers serving sweat glands (they use ACh)

What receptors does NE bind to?

α- or β-receptors

Where do you find the following enzymes?

MAO

In presynaptic terminals

COMT

In adjacent astrocytes as well as in postsynaptic terminal

Where is Epi mainly secreted?

Adrenal medulla

Where is dopamine mainly released?

Striatum (putamen and caudate)

What is its relationship to prolactin?	Inhibits its secretion (aka prolactin-inhibitory factor)
Where is dopamine predominantly located?	Midbrain neurons (~80% is located in the basal ganglia)
What metabolizes dopamine?	MAO and COMT
What occurs when dopamine binds to the following receptors?	
D_1 receptor	Activates adenylate cyclase via a G_s protein
D_2 receptor	Inhibits adenylate cyclase via a G_i protein
How is the dopamine signal terminated?	Reuptake into the presynaptic terminal
What receptor type may be more prevalent in schizophrenics?	D_2 receptors
What is serotonin derived from?	Tryptophan
Where are high concentrations of serotonin found?	Brain stem
What is serotonin converted into by the pineal gland?	Melatonin
Where is serotonin primarily synthesized?	Raphe nucleus; projects widely to forebrain and brain stem
What is histamine derived from?	Histidine
Where is histamine present as a neurotransmitter?	Hypothalamus

NEUROMUSCULAR JUNCTION

What is the neuromuscular junction (NMJ)?	Synapse between an axon from a motor neuron and skeletal muscle
What is the neurotransmitter in the NMJ?	Acetylcholine (ACh)
What type of receptor is on the postsynaptic membrane?	Nicotinic receptor
What enzyme catalyzes the formation of ACh in the presynaptic terminal?	Choline acetyltransferase

What are the constituent pieces that are used to produce ACh?

Acetyl coenzyme A (CoA) and choline

What type of channel is the nicotinic receptor on the muscle end plate (postsynaptic membrane)?

Ligand-gated channel

What ion(s) changes permeability with binding of ACh to its receptor on the motor end plate?

Na^+ (primarily) and K^+

How does depolarization of the motor end-plate spread?

Local currents cause depolarization in adjacent muscle

What degrades the ACh in the synaptic cleft and on the motor end plate?

Acetylcholinesterase (AChE); this is the only transmitter that is degraded extracellularly

Why is degradation of ACh in the synaptic cleft and on the motor end plate necessary?

Permanent binding would cause permanent depolarization of the motor end plate and maintain muscle contraction (e.g., tetany)

What are the actions of the following agents on the neuromuscular junction?

Botulinus toxin

Blocks release of ACh from the presynaptic terminal

Curare

Competes with ACh for receptors on the motor end plate

Hemicholinium

Blocks reuptake of choline into the presynaptic terminal

Neostigmine

Inhibits acetylcholinesterase

What are the effects on neuromuscular transmission of the following agents?

Botulinus toxin

Total blockade of neuromuscular transmission

Curare

Decreases the size of the end-plate potential (EPP)

Hemicholinium

Prolongs and enhances the action of ACh at the muscle end plate

Neostigmine

Depletes the ACh store of the presynaptic terminal

What is the pathophysiologic basis of myasthenia gravis?

Presence of ACh receptor antibodies decreases the number of binding sites on the muscle end plate

SKELETAL AND SMOOTH MUSCLE

What are the components of a skeletal muscle fiber?

1. Bundles of myofibrils
2. Surrounding sarcoplasmic reticulum (SR)
3. Transverse (T) tubules

What is a sarcomere?

Myofibril unit

Identify the labeled items in the following figure:

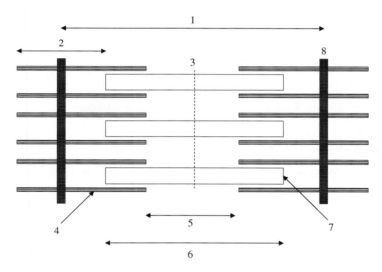

Figure 1.5   The Sarcomere.

1. Sarcomere
2. I band
3. M line
4. Thin filament
5. H band
6. A band
7. Thick filament
8. Z line

How are the filaments in a sarcomere arranged in skeletal muscle?

Longitudinally

What are thick filaments made up of?

Myosin protein

What are the components of myosin?

Six polypeptide chains: two heavy chains and four light chains

What are thin filaments made up of?	Actin, tropomyosin, and troponin
What are the components of troponin and what are their functions?	Troponin C: Binds Ca^{2+} and allows interaction of actin and myosin
	Troponin I: Inhibits interaction of actin and myosin
	Troponin T: Attaches troponin to tropomyosin
	(Remember: C = Ca^{2+}, I = inhibits, T = troponin)
What are the functions of the sarcoplasmic reticulum (SR)?	Maintains low intracellular $[Ca^{2+}]$, stores and releases Ca^{2+} for use in the excitation-contraction coupling
What is the function of the T tubule?	To deliver the action potential to the SR. These are continuous with the extracellular space
How are the SR and T tubule connected?	At terminal cisternae
How is Ca^{2+} stored in the SR?	Loosely bound to calsequestrin
How is Ca^{2+} transported into the SR?	Ca^{2+}-ATPase pump on the SR membrane
How does Ca^{2+} exit the SR?	Via the ryanodine receptor (Ca^{2+} channel)

Describe the steps in excitation-contraction coupling that permit the cross-bridge cycle for muscle contraction:

Action potential occurs

↓

T tubules depolarize

↓

Ca^{2+} channels open on SR membrane

↓

Intracellular $[Ca^{2+}]$ increases

↓

Ca^{2+} bind to troponin C

↓

Troponin undergoes conformational change moving tropomyosin from the myosin-binding site on actin

↓

Cross-bridge cycle occurs

Describe the steps in the cross-bridge cycle that leads to muscle contraction:

Myosin has no ATP bound and is tightly attached to actin

↓

ATP binds to myosin causing a conformational change that releases actin

↓

Hydrolysis of ATP into ADP and inorganic phosphate (Pi) displace myosin toward the plus end of actin

↓

Myosin binds to a new site on actin, which generates the power for contraction

↓

ADP is released, returning myosin to its tightly bound state

What limits the cross-bridge cycle?

Ca^{2+} being bound to troponin C and exposing the myosin-binding sites on actin

What causes muscle relaxation?

Reuptake of Ca^{2+} by the SR

What would occur if the intracellular $[Ca^{2+}]$ remained high in a skeletal muscle cell?

The muscle would not be able to relax (e.g., tetany)

What is an isometric contraction?

Force is generated without muscle shortening

What is an isotonic contraction?

Muscle fiber shortens at a constant afterload

What is afterload?

Load that the muscle contracts against

What is passive tension?

Tension developed by the muscle as it is stretched to different lengths. This is a consequence of the physical elements of the myocyte.

What is total tension?

Tension developed by the muscle when it contracts at different lengths

What is active tension?

The difference between total tension and passive tension

What is active tension proportional to?

The number of cross-bridges formed in the muscle

When is tension maximum?	When there is maximum overlap of thick and thin filaments permitting the most cross-bridges to form
Why does active tension decrease when the muscle is stretched maximally?	The number of cross-bridges that can form is smaller than when the muscle is at tension maximum
What happens to the velocity of shortening in a muscle as the afterload increases?	Decreases
What are the components of smooth muscle?	Thick filaments and thin filaments
Are there sarcomeres in smooth muscle?	No
Is there troponin in smooth muscle?	No
The lack of troponin in smooth muscle leads to what histological consequence?	Smooth muscle does not have striations
What are the types of smooth muscle?	Multiunit, single-unit, and vascular
Which type is most common?	Single-unit
Which type has a high degree of electrical coupling between cells?	Single-unit
What type has spontaneous (*pacemaker*) activity?	Single-unit
What type is densely innervated?	Multiunit
Do multiunit smooth muscle units coordinate?	No, they behave separately
What properties does vascular smooth muscle exhibit?	Mix of multiunit and single-unit properties
What regulates excitation-contraction coupling in smooth muscle?	Ca^{2+} (there is no troponin!)
What are the mechanisms by which intracellular $[Ca^{2+}]$ can be increased in smooth muscle?	1. Depolarization of the cell membrane opens voltage-gated Ca^{2+} channels 2. SR may release additional Ca^{2+} with depolarization 3. SR can be stimulated by hormones and neurotransmitters to release Ca^{2+} via IP_3-gated Ca^{2+} channels

Describe excitation-contraction coupling in smooth muscle:

Intracellular $[Ca^{2+}]$ increases
$\downarrow$
Ca^{2+} binds to calmodulin activating myosin light-chain kinase
$\downarrow$
Myosin is phosphorylated and binds to actin
$\downarrow$
Shortening occurs

What causes relaxation in smooth muscle?

Dephosphorylation of myosin

CLINICAL VIGNETTES

A researcher has found a new drug, but to be most effective, it has to get across the lipid bilayer. What two characteristics of the drug can help to encourage transcellular movement?

Either increasing the oil/water partition coefficient or decreasing the overall size of the molecule.

A young man is inadvertently given a dose of tetrodotoxin and his excitable cells are no longer able to generate action potentials, how did this occur?

Voltage-sensitive Na^+ channels are blocked and action potentials cannot be produced

Some of a patient's blood is collected and an unknown solution is added to the sample. When the technician views the slide, all of the red blood cells (RBCs) have lysed. What is the osmolarity of the added solution relative to the patient's sample?

Hypotonic

A young woman is poisoned by a jealous friend with an agent that inhibits her cell's Na^+-K^+-ATPase. What will happen to the concentrations of intracellular Na^+, K^+, and Ca^{2+}?

Increase in intracellular Na^+, decrease in intracellular K^+, and increase in intracellular Ca^{2+} from decreased Na^+ gradient

A 71-year-old man comes in with a shuffling gait, a blank facial expression and a severe intention tremor. You recognize these symptoms as Parkinson syndrome. What is the underlying pathology?

Degeneration of dopaminergic neurons in the substantia nigra and pars compacta that utilize D_2 receptors.
    In the subcortical circuit that these neurons are involved in, the dopamine aids in the initiation of movement related tasks, without it, motor activities tend to be difficult to *begin*.

A 26-year-old man comes in with a low sodium value after he had been drinking buckets and buckets of beer without eating anything for the past several weeks (a condition called beer potomania). Being a new intern, you mistakenly decide to infuse a high sodium solution to resuscitate. You drastically overcorrect. What happens to the tonicity of the blood? What happens to the body's water balance?

With the infusion of a hypertonic solution, intravascular fluid will become hypertonic. With this change, water will flow toward the area of high tonicity leading to cellular shrinkage.

While this causes problems systemically, this is especially dangerous in the brain where this rapid fluid flux can lead to the loss of myelin from around the axons of neurons, a process called central pontine myelinolysis.

A researcher is studying muscular contraction and has set up an experiment whereby some muscle fibers are constantly stimulated. Once he begins the stimulation he notes that the muscles enter a state of tetanic contraction. What ion is responsible for this and what would its concentration be inside the muscle cells?

Ca^{2+} is responsible for the tetany. It would be at very high levels due to constant release by the sarcoplasmic reticulum (SR). The constant stimulation the muscle fibers are receiving demands continuous Ca^{++} release and it is not being reaccumulated by the SR.

Detectives get a call about a shooting. When they arrive on scene, they find a young man has been shot and killed. As they are inspecting the body for clues, it is noted to be in a rigid state. What is the physiologic basis for this state?

Rigor mortis is due to the lack of adenosine triphosphate (ATP). After a person dies, the body is no longer able to regenerate ATP. ATP is used to release myosin from actin thus in its absence, skeletal muscle fibers remain tightly bound, producing a rigid state.

CHAPTER 2

Neurophysiology

AUTONOMIC NERVOUS SYSTEM

What are the two *structural* divisions of the human nervous system?

1. Central nervous system
2. Peripheral nervous system

What are the two *functional* divisions of the human nervous system?

1. Somatic nervous system
2. Autonomic nervous system (ANS)

What is the function of the somatic nervous system?

Innervates skeletal muscle; largely under voluntary control

What is the function of the ANS?

Maintenance of homeostasis through involuntary coordination of glandular, cardiac, and smooth muscle activity throughout the body

What are the constituent parts of the ANS?

Enteric nervous system, sympathetic nervous system (SNS), and parasympathetic nervous system (PNS)

Generally speaking, what is the function of each part of the ANS?

Enteric nervous system

Coordination of various gut functions (motility, secretion, etc) (see Chap. 6)

Sympathetic nervous system

"Fight or flight" response. Coordinates the body's response to stressors.

Parasympathetic nervous system

"Rest and digest" response. Coordinates the process of energy conservation and replenishment.

Where is the anatomic origin of SNS?

Intermediolateral cell column of the spinal cord between segments T1 to L3 (e.g., thoracolumbar)

Where is the anatomic origin of the PNS?

Nuclei of cranial nerves (CN) III, VII, IX, and X and spinal cord segments S2 to S4 (e.g., craniosacral spinal cord)

What type(s) of neurotransmitter(s) and receptors are present in the *preganglionic* fibers of the PNS and SNS?

PNS and SNS preganglionic neurons use ACh as the neurotransmitter and nicotinic receptors for transmission

Is the neurotransmitter/receptor combination used at the preganglionic synapse the same as that used at the neuromuscular junction (NMJ)?

No, while these receptors are nAChR (nicotinic Acetylcholine receptors) they differ from those at the NMJ. The nicotinic subunits here have a different subunit makeup allowing for differences in pharmacologic influences

Describe the axon length for the PNS and SNS in the following locations:

	PNS	SNS
Preganglionic nerve axon	Long	Short
Postganglionic nerve axon	Short	Long

Anatomically, where do most preganglionic sympathetic fibers synapse?

Either at the paravertebral chain ganglion, or at collateral ganglia that follow large vessels in the abdomen (celiac, superior mesenteric, etc)

Anatomically, where do most preganglionic parasympathetic fibers synapse?

In microscopic ganglia associated with the target organs

What receptor types are primarily used at the effector organs of the PNS and SNS? What are their respective neurotransmitters?

PNS: all receptors are muscarinic and ACh is the neurotransmitter

SNS: α_1, α_2, β_1, or β_2; the primary neurotransmitter is norepinephrine (NE)

There is an exception to the above rule regarding the SNS. What is it?

Sweat glands have muscarinic receptors. The associated postganglionic SNS neurons release ACh.

What is unique about the adrenal medulla?

It is a specialized SNS ganglion where preganglionic fibers synapse directly with the effector organ (chromaffin cells)

What does SNS stimulation of chromaffin cells induce?

Secretion of epinephrine (Epi; 80%) and NE (20%) into the circulation

What is the purpose of releasing adrenal hormones into the circulation?

These substances activate organs that receive little innervation (fat cells, hepatocytes etc) allowing them to assist in the stress response

What are the SNS receptor types in the following locations and what are their effects?

Heart

SA node	β_1: increased pacemaker activity
AV node	β_1: increased conduction velocity
Myocardium	β_1: increased contractility

Vascular smooth muscle

Skin and splanchnic circuits	α_1 and α_2: constriction
Skeletal muscle and pulmonary circuits	β_2: dilation
Peripheral veins	α_1: constriction
	β_2: dilation

Eye

Ciliary muscle	β_1: relaxes muscle (for far vision)
Radial muscle	α_1: muscle contraction $\rightarrow$ dilates pupil

Bladder

Detrusor muscle	β_2: relaxes
Bladder sphincter	α_1: constricts

Bronchioles

Bronchial muscle	β_2: dilates smooth muscle
Bronchial glands	α_1: inhibits secretion
	β_2: stimulates secretion

Gastrointestinal tract

Sphincters	α_1: constricts
Secretion	α_2: inhibition
Motility	$\alpha_1, \alpha_2, \beta_2$: decrease

Kidney β_1: increase renin secretion

Male sex organs	α_1: ejaculation
Sweat glands	Muscarinic: increase sweat production
Adipose tissue	β_1, β_3: increase lipolysis

For which of the above SNS locations is there no corresponding PNS innervation?

Vascular smooth muscle, kidney, sweat glands, fat cells, and liver

What is the mechanism of action for the following receptor types?

α_1	Inositol 1,4,5-triphosphate (IP_3) formation and increased intracellular $[Ca^{2+}]$
α_2	Adenylate cyclase inhibition and decreased cyclic adenosine monophosphate (cAMP)
β_1	Adenylate cyclase activation and increased cAMP
β_2	Adenylate cyclase activation and increased cAMP
Nicotinic	Ion channel for Na^+ and K^+
Muscarinic	Heart (sinoatrial [SA] node): adenylate cyclase inhibition
	Smooth muscle and glands: IP_3 formation and increased intracellular $[Ca^{2+}]$

What is the effect on the ANS of the following pharmacologic agents?

ACh	Nicotinic and muscarinic agonist
Albuterol	β_2 Agonist
Atropine	Muscarinic antagonist
Butoxamine	β_2 Antagonist
Carbachol	Nicotinic and muscarinic agonist
Clonidine	α_2 Agonist
Curare	Nicotinic antagonist
Dobutamine	β_1 Agonist
Hexamethonium	Nicotinic antagonist (ganglion only)
Isoproterenol	β_1 and β_2 agonist
Metoprolol (at therapeutic doses)	β_1 Antagonist
Muscarine	Muscarinic agonist
Nicotine	Nicotinic agonist
NE	α_1 and β_1 agonist
Phenoxybenzamine	$\alpha_{1,2}$ Antagonist
Phentolamine	$\alpha_{1,2}$ Antagonist
Phenylephrine	α_1 Agonist
Prazosin	α_1 Antagonist
Propranolol	β_1 and β_2 antagonist
Yohimbine	α_2 Antagonist

What autonomic centers are located
in the following areas?

Medulla	Respiratory; swallowing, coughing, and vomiting; and vasomotor
Pons	Pneumotaxic
Midbrain	Micturition
Hypothalamus	Regulation of food and liquid intake and temperature regulation

SENSORY SYSTEMS

What four qualities of sensation must be encoded for effective transmission?

1. Modality
2. Location
3. Intensity
4. Duration

What is a sensory receptor?

A specialized cell that transduces physical environmental stimuli into neural signals

What types of cells are usually sensory receptors?

Specialized epithelial and neuronal cells

What is meant by "receptive field"?

Area on the body that changes the firing rate of its sensory neuron when stimulated

What is the field called if it increases the firing rate?

Excitatory

What is the field called if it decreases the firing rate?

Inhibitory

A sensory receptor must transmit its findings back to the CNS for interpretation. How does the CNS differentiate between an AP (action potential) from a retinal cell and an AP from a somatosensory cell?

The receptors are simple transducers, each converting a different type of energy into electrical impulses. These impulses follow defined pathways into the CNS and relay on specific nuclei. These pathways define how sensory perception is recognized.

For an example of this, think about rubbing your eyes. That pressure is always perceived as flashes of light.

How are afferent neurons of the sensory systems classified?

By diameter (roman numerals I-IV) and conduction velocity (A and C)

Give the relative size of the following sensory neuron classifications:

I	Largest
II	Medium
III	Small
IV	Smallest

Give the relative conduction velocity of the following sensory neuron classifications:

Aα	Fastest
Aβ	Medium
Aδ	Medium
C	Slowest

Describe the series of events that occur in sensory transduction.

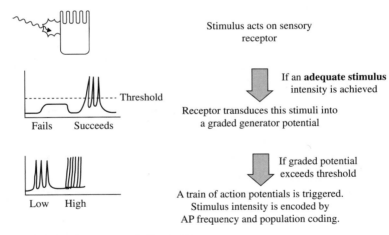

Stimulus acts on sensory receptor

If an **adequate stimulus** intensity is achieved

Receptor transduces this stimuli into a graded generator potential

If graded potential exceeds threshold

A train of action potentials is triggered. Stimulus intensity is encoded by AP frequency and population coding.

Figure 2.1   Sensory transduction sequence.

What effect does intensity of the stimulus have on the receptor potential generated?

Larger stimuli create larger graded potentials (e.g., receptor potential)

What direction does the current usually flow when sensory receptor channels open?

Positive inward flow, depolarizing the cell

What is an exception to this flow direction?

Photoreceptors: stimulation decreases inward current and hyperpolarizes the membrane

As seen in Fig. 2.1, how does the body encode intensity changes in sensory stimuli?

Primarily with frequency coding; greater intensity leads to a higher frequency. Also with population coding; a greater number of receptors will be triggered by a stimulus of increasing intensity.

What is sensory adaptation?

The dynamic change in the frequency of triggered AP's with a static stimuli; this occurs at the level of the receptor

What types of adaptation do sensory receptors exhibit?

Tonic (slowly adapting) and phasic (rapidly adapting)

Which type of sensory adaptation detects the beginning of (onset) and the end of (offset) of a stimulus?

Phasic

What type of sensory adaptation responds consistently to prolonged stimuli?

Tonic

What type of sensory adaptation detects steady stimuli?

Tonic

What happens to action potential frequency in phasic receptors with constant stimulation?

Decreases

Label the three types of adaptation seen below:

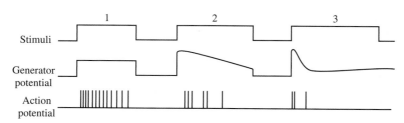

Figure 2.2   Adaptation.

1. No Adaptation, also called tonic adaptation
2. Slowly adapting sensory neurons
3. Rapidly adapting sensory neurons, also called phasic adaptation

What is the location of the following structures?

First-order neurons

Dorsal root ganglia

Second-order neurons

Spinal cord or brain stem (depending on system)

Third-order neurons

Thalamus (relay nuclei)

What goes on beyond the relay nucleus?	Extensively overlapping cortical circuitry that interprets external stimuli and relays information throughout the cortex

Somatosensory System

What sensations are perceived by the somatosensory system?	Touch, movement, and position, as well as temperature, and pain
What two anatomical pathways does the somatosensory system use?	1. Dorsal-column system 2. Anterolateral system

What sensations are detected by the following systems?

Dorsal-column system	Touch, vibration, and proprioception
Anterolateral system	Temperature and pain

What path does sensory information take in the dorsal-column system?

Receptors with cell bodies in the dorsal root ganglia receive stimulus (first order)
↓
Signal ascends to the nucleus gracilis and nucleus cuneatus in medulla (still first order)
↓
Signal crosses the midline and ascends to enter contralateral thalamus (second order)
↓
Signal ascends to the somatosensory cortex (third order)

What path does sensory information take in the anterolateral system?

Receptors with cell bodies in the dorsal root ganglia receive stimulus (first order)
↓
Signal crosses the midline and enters the anterolateral quadrant of the spinal cord (second order)
↓
Signal ascends to contralateral thalamus (still second order)
↓
Signal sent to somatosensory cortex (third order)

What are the major differences between the two systems with respect to the anatomy of the ascending information?

Dorsal columns don't cross midline until the medulla; anterolateral system crosses at the level of the peripheral nerve

Ascending information in dorsal columns carried by first-order neuron; in the anterolateral system, it is carried by the second-order neuron

What are the tracts of Lissauer?

These are found at the dorsal root where the anterolateral system enters the spinal cord. They allow for fibers to move vertically one or two segments before synapsing.

What is another name for the sensory cortex?

Sensory homunculus

How is the homunculus arranged?

Upside down (face most lateral, with feet and genitals inside the central sulcus)

Why are the face, hands, and genital regions of the homunculus so large?

They possess the highest density of nerve fibers

What are the types of mechanoreceptors that detect touch and pressure?

Meissner corpuscle

Merkel disk

Pacinian corpuscle

Ruffini corpuscle

What sensation is encoded by the following mechanoreceptors?

    Meissner corpuscle

Velocity

    Merkel disk

Pressure–small receptive field

    Pacinian corpuscle

Vibration

    Ruffini corpuscle

Pressure–large receptive field

Which types of mechanoreceptors demonstrate phasic adaptation?

Meissner and Pacinian corpuscles

Which types of mechanoreceptors demonstrate tonic adaptation?

Merkel disks and Ruffini corpuscles

What is nociception?

Detection and perception of noxious stimuli (e.g., pain)

What types of receptors detect pain?

No specialized receptors; pain is detected by free nerve endings

What triggers pain receptors?	Any excessive application of energy (chemical, thermal, or mechanical)
Where are pain receptors located?	Skin, muscle, and viscera
What two pathways does visceral pain stimulate?	1. Visceral afferent fibers ascend with sympathetic nerves 2. Referred to the skin in a dermatomal fashion
Explain referred pain:	Afferent pain fibers serving the viscera enter the spinal cord at particular levels. Since the body is not used to visceral pain, it confuses those stimuli with dermatomal pain from the same spinal root.
What fibers carry fast pain signals?	Group III
What fibers carry slow pain signals?	C fibers
Opiates inhibit the release of what neurotransmitter for nociception?	Substance P

VISION

In the image below, label the numbered portions of the eye.

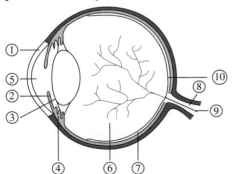

1. Cornea
2. Iris
3. Lens
4. Ciliary body
5. Aqueous humor
6. Vitreous humor
7. Retina
8. Optic nerve
9. Central vessels of the retina
10. Fovea

Figure 2.3   The eye.

What is the function of the lens?	Focuses light onto the retina
What is the condition called when the curvature of the lens is not uniform?	Astigmatism

What structure produces aqueous humor?

Ciliary epithelium covering the surface of the ciliary body

How does aqueous humor drain?

Via the canal of Schlemm

What conditions are described by the following?

    Lens focuses light onto the retina

Emmetropia (this is normal)

    Lens focuses light in front of the retina

Myopia (nearsighted)

    Lens focuses light behind the retina

Hyperopia (farsighted)

What is accommodation?

Focusing of light by the lens

How does accommodation occur?

The smooth muscle of the ciliary body contracts to focus the lens

What is presbyopia?

Loss of accommodation due to stiffening of the lens

Identify the labeled cell types of the retina in the image below.

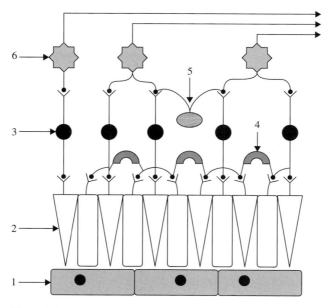

Figure 2.4 Retina.

1. Pigment epithelial cells
2. Receptors (rods and cones)
3. Bipolar cells
4. Horizontal cells
5. Amacrine cells
6. Ganglion cells

What are the functions of the following cell types?

Pigment epithelial cells	Absorbs light reflecting off retina preventing it from interfering with retinal phototransduction
Photoreceptors (rods and cones)	Convert 11-*cis* retinal to all-*trans* retinal (photoisomerization) initiating phototransduction
Horizontal cells	Form local circuits with bipolar cells in the outer plexiform layer
Amacrine cells	Form local circuits with bipolar cells in the inner plexiform layer

Identify the following characteristics of rods and cones (e.g., photoreceptors):

	Cones	Rods
Acuity	High	Low
Type of light sensitive to	High-intensity	Low-intensity
Color vision	Present	Absent
Dark adaptation	Fast	Slow

Why do rods have lower acuity compared to cones?	Many rods synapse on a single bipolar cell, whereas only a few cones synapse on a single bipolar cell
What is rhodopsin?	Visual pigment found in the photoreceptors that absorbs photons of light energy
What are the molecular components of rhodopsin?	Opsin (protein) and retinal (light-absorbing vitamin A analogue)
How does rhodopsin differ between rods and cones?	Rods have one type of opsin. Cones have three types: red, green, and blue.
What conformation is retinal normally in?	11-*cis* retinal
What happens when light hits the retina?	Photoreceptors absorb individual photons and 11-*cis* retinal is converted to all-*trans* retinal (photoisomerization)
What is required to regenerate 11-*cis* retinal?	Vitamin A
When *not* exposed to light, is the photoreceptor depolarized or hyperpolarized?	Depolarized. A constant inward Na^+ current maintains depolarization.

What is the consequence of photoreceptor tonic depolarization?	Tonic release of glutamate (inhibitory neurotransmitter) onto the bipolar cells
After a photon of light is absorbed by rhodopsin, leading to photoisomerization, what changes?	Opsin binds to *transducin*; activating it. That shuts down the cGMP cascade that has maintained depolarization of the photoreceptor. As a result, the cell hyperpolarizes.
How does photoreceptor hyperpolarization lead to stimulatory output to the brain?	Cell hyperpolarization inhibits the release of glutamate. Now the bipolar cell can fire an excitatory-graded potential.
What is the fovea?	Area on the retina where acuity is the highest
Are there rods present in the fovea?	No
What is the relationship of cones to bipolar cells in the fovea?	1:1
How is an image formed on the retina?	The image is inverted and reversed with respect to the object
What is the optic disk?	A feature seen on opthalmoscopic examination; it is the location where the axons from the ganglion cells converge to form the optic nerve
What is the blind spot?	Correlates to the location of the optic disk; approximately 15° off center where no rods or cones are present
What is the optic chiasm?	Location where fifty percent of the nerve fibers cross the midline to form the contralateral optic tract
Fibers from which hemiretina, nasal or temporal, cross the midline in the optic chiasm?	Nasal hemiretina
The nasal hemiretina sees which portion of the visual field?	The temporal visual field
Where do the nerve fibers that form the right optic tract originate?	Right temporal hemiretina and left nasal hemiretina

Describe the visual defect present with the following lesions in the optic pathway:

Right optic-nerve transection	Right eye is totally blind
Optic chiasm transaction/compression	Bitemporal hemianopia
Optic tract	Homonymous hemianopia
Left Meyer loop transection	Right upper quadrantanopia
Transection of right-visual radiation to cuneus	Left lower quadrantanopia
Left visual cortex (occipital lobe)	Right hemianopia with macular sparing

Where is the primary visual cortex located?

In the Brodmann area 17, located principally on the sides of the calcarine fissure

For what part of the visual field are most of the optic fibers carrying information?

Ninety percent of optic nerve fibers carry information from the central 30° of the visual field

What is the consensual light reflex?

A reflex whereby shining a light in one eye normally leads to constriction of both pupils

What is the neural pathway for the consensual light reflex?

Light entering one eye is detected by CN II, some of which is relayed to the pretectal nucleus which communicates with the contralateral pretectal nucleus through the posterior commissure. Information is sent to the Edinger-Westphal nucleus which then relays information to the ciliary body through CN III.

Define nystagmus:

It is a repetitive, tremor-like oscillating movement of the eyes

AUDITORY AND VESTIBULAR SYSTEM

The outer ear is responsible for what?

Collecting and directing sound waves toward the tympanic membrane

What is the function of tympanic membrane?

It vibrates in response to pressure changes produced by sound waves on its external surface and imparts its motions to the manubrium of the malleus

What are the auditory ossicles?	The three bones located in the middle ear: malleus, incus, and stapes
What is the purpose of the ossicles?	They act as a series of levers to amplify the vibrations of the tympanic membrane and direct them toward the oval window
What is the purpose of the oval and the round window?	The oval window is the connection between the middle and inner ear that permits entry of sound waves; the round window allows the energy that enters the inner ear to dissipate.
What makes up the inner ear?	Bony labyrinth (a series of channels in the petrous portion of the temporal bone) and membranous labyrinth (duplicates the shape of the bony channels)
What makes up the bony labyrinth?	Semicircular canals, cochlea, and vestibule
What are the fluids in the inner ear and where are they located?	Perilymph is the fluid outside the ducts and endolymph is the fluid inside the ducts
What ion is predominant in the inner ear fluids?	Perilymph: Na^+ Endolymph: K^+

Identify the labeled structures of the inner ear in the figure below:

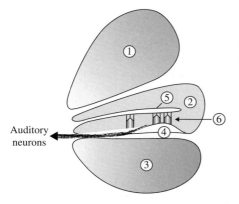

1. Scala vestibuli
2. Scala media
3. Scala tympani
4. Basilar membrane
5. Tectorial membrane
6. Organ of Corti

Auditory neurons

Figure 2.5 Inner ear.

How is sound transmitted to the brain?

Sound waves are directed to the auditory canal by the outer ear

↓

Transformed by the tympanic membrane and auditory ossicles into movements of the footplate of the stapes, which rests on the oval window

↓

Pressure changes transmitted by the stapes causes waves in the perilymph of the inner ear

↓

The basilar membrane moves in response to the perilymph fluid wave; this movement affects overlying hair cells which transduce sound into neural input

What are hair cells?

The receptor cells for auditory stimuli and acceleration (both angular and linear) of the head

Where are hair cells located?

On the basilar membrane of the cochlea (audition) and vestibular organ (acceleration)

What is the organ of Corti?

The structure located on the basilar membrane of the cochlea that contains the hair cells, which are the auditory receptors

How is sound transduced by the organ of Corti?

Fluid waves in the scala tympani cause vibration of basilar membrane; the cilia on basilar membrane bump against the overlying tectorial membrane

↓

Cilia bend, which changes the cation conductance of the hair cell membrane

↓

Direction of bend causes depolarization or hyperpolarization depending on whether cation channels are opened or closed

↓

Oscillating potential (cochlear microphonic potential) generated

What frequencies of sound are best detected in the following locations?

Apex of the basilar membrane (furthest from oval window) — Low frequencies

Base of the basilar membrane (nearest the oval window) — High frequencies

What is unique about the auditory nerve fiber's path?

Fibers may be crossed or uncrossed, which means that once nerve fibers enter the brain, all higher levels receive input from both ears

How do you perform the following tests?

Weber test

A 512 Hz tuning fork is struck and the handle placed on the patient's head in the midline. The patient indicates whether he or she hears or feels the sound in the right ear, the left ear, or in the middle of the forehead.

Rinne test

A 512 Hz tuning fork is struck and its handle placed on the patient's mastoid tip. The patient is asked if he or she hears a sound and if so, indicates when the sound is no longer heard. At this point, the tines of the tuning fork are placed in front of the external auditory meatus of the same ear and the patient is asked if a sound is still heard. This is then repeated for the patient's other ear.

How do the following characteristics differ in the Rinne and Weber test to distinguish conduction deafness from nerve deafness?

	Rinne	Weber
Normal hearing	Air conduction > bone conduction	Hears sound in the middle
Conduction deafness	Bone conduction > air conduction	Sound is louder in diseased ear
Sensorineural deafness	Air conduction > bone conduction	Sound is louder in normal ear

Which structures in the ear are concerned with equilibrium?

Semicircular canals, utricle, and saccule of the inner ear

Which direction of acceleration do the following detect?

Semicircular canal	Rotational
Utricle	Linear and horizontal
Saccule	Linear and vertical

What occurs when the stereocilia of the hair cell:

Bend toward the kinocilium?	The hair cell depolarizes
Bend away from the kinocilium?	The hair cell hyperpolarizes

TASTE AND OLFACTION

What is involved in the act of tasting food and beverages?

1. Direct chemical stimulation of taste buds
2. Stimulation of olfactory receptors by vapors from food
3. Stimulation of chemical-sensitive and somatosensory free nerve endings of the trigeminal and other nerves in the mucous membranes of the oral and nasal cavities

What are taste buds?

Papillae on the surface of the tongue, as well as the pharynx

What is the role of microvilli on taste buds?

Increases the surface area to bind taste chemicals

What types of papillae are there and where are they located?

Fungiform: anterior two-thirds of tongue

Circumvallate: posterior one-third of tongue

Foliate: posterior one-third of tongue

What are the five basic taste qualities?

1. Sweet
2. Salty
3. Sour
4. Bitter
5. Umami

What tastes do the various papillae discriminate?

Fungiform: salty and sweet

Circumvallate: sour and bitter

Foliate: sour and bitter

What transduction processes are involved with each of the basic taste qualities?

Sweet: Compounds bind to G-protein-coupled receptors resulting in decreased K^+ conductance and depolarization.

Salty: Sodium channels in the apical membranes of taste receptor cells allow influx of Na^+ ions resulting in depolarization of the cell.

Sour: Acidic compounds cause increased H^+ concentration resulting in depolarization of receptor cells either by direct proton influx through sodium channels or by blocking conductance of pH-sensitive apical K^+ channels.

Bitter: Compounds often found in toxic substances. Receptor cells use both ligand-gated channels and G-protein-coupled receptors that result in release of calcium ions from internal stores.

Umami: Receptors respond to amino acids. Ionotropic glutamate receptor stimulates Na^+ and Ca^{++} entry into the cell.

The fibers that innervate the following regions originate in which CN?

Anterior two-thirds of tongue

CN VII (chorda tympani)

Posterior one-third of tongue

CN IX (glossopharyngeal)

Back of throat/epiglottis

CN X (vagus)

What is the pathway for taste?

CN VII, IX, and X enter the medulla and travel caudally to the solitary tract where they synapse on second-order taste neurons in the solitary nucleus; fibers ascend from there ipsilaterally to ventral posteromedial nucleus of the thalamus and onto the taste cortex

Which CN mediates olfaction?

CN I

What role does CN V play on olfaction?

It innervates the olfactory epithelium, which detects noxious or painful stimuli

What structure do the olfactory nerves pass through that, when damaged, can induce hyposmia or anosmia?

Cribriform plate

How are olfactory receptors unique?

They are the only neurons that are replaced throughout a person's life

Which part of the brain are olfactory receptor neurons considered part of?

They are a direct part of the ipsilateral telencephalon and do not relay in the thalamus

Describe the transduction of olfaction:

Olfactory receptor neurons bind odorant molecules

↓

Activate G proteins

↓

Activate adenylate cyclase

↓

Increase intracellular [cAMP]

↓

Na^+ channels opened

↓

Depolarization of receptor potential

MOTOR NEUROPHYSIOLOGY

For further review, see the neuromuscular junction section in Chap. 1.

What types of muscle fibers are there?   Extrafusal and intrafusal

Which type generates the force for contraction?   Extrafusal fibers

Which type monitors muscle tension?   Intrafusal fibers

What are the innervations for the following?

Extrafusal fibers α-Motoneurons

Intrafusal fibers γ-Motoneurons

Define the following:

Motor unit   Single motoneuron and the muscle fibers it innervates

Small motoneuron   Motoneuron that innervates only a few muscle fibers

Large motoneuron   Motoneuron that innervates many muscle fibers

Motoneuron pool   Collection of motoneurons that innervate the muscle fibers of the same muscle

For small and large motoneurons identify the following characteristics:	Small Motoneuron	Large Motoneuron
Force generation	Small	Large
Threshold level	Low	High
Firing time	Fast	Slow

How is muscle contraction increased?

By recruitment of additional motor units

What is the size principle with respect to force generation in motor units?

As motor units are recruited, more motoneurons become involved, which generate more tension

How is the spinal circuit arranged?

The α-motor neuron receives three inputs:

1. Upper motor neuron pathways
2. Spinal interneurons (involved in reflex and central pattern generation)
3. Sensory input from muscle

What type of muscle sensors are there and what do they detect?

Muscle spindles: detect changes in muscle length (both dynamic and static)

Golgi tendon organs: detect muscle tension

Pacinian corpuscles: detect vibration

Free nerve endings: detect noxious stimuli

What are muscle spindles?

Intrafusal fibers that have been encapsulated in sheaths and are connected in parallel with extrafusal fibers

What is meant by "intrafusal fiber?"

Specialized muscle fibers that are arranged in *parallel* to the extrafusal (force generating) fibers to provide feedback about muscle length/tension changes

What types of intrafusal fibers can be in muscle spindles?

Nuclear bag fibers and nuclear chain fibers

Which type is more numerous?

Nuclear chain fibers

What do the following fibers detect?

Nuclear chain fibers

Changes in muscle length

Nuclear bag fibers

Dynamic changes in muscle length (e.g., velocity)

What is the innervation for nuclear chain fibers?	Group II afferent fibers
What is the innervation for nuclear bag fibers?	Group Ia afferent fibers
What stimulus is detected by muscle spindles?	Muscle stretch (e.g., lengthened)
What is the response of nuclear bag fibers to stimulation?	Group Ia afferent fibers stimulate α-motoneurons in the spinal cord, which causes contraction in the muscle (e.g., shortening)
What role do γ-motoneurons play in the muscle fiber reflex?	These ensure that the muscle spindle will be primed (set to the correct length) so that they can appropriately respond to either voluntary or involuntary changes in muscle length
How is the ratio of intrafusal: extrafusal fibers different in the hand versus the quadriceps?	Higher in the hand; just as the hand has many more motoneurons to allow for finer control, it has many more muscle spindles to provide feedback during movement
Where are the Golgi tendon organs located?	These are encapsulated inside muscle tendons; these are arranged in *series* with the extrafusal fibers. These provide information about the force of muscle contraction.
What are the major muscle reflex types and how many synapses does each use?	Stretch reflex: monosynaptic Golgi tendon reflex: disynaptic Flexor-withdrawal reflex: polysynaptic
Describe the stretch reflex:	Muscle is stretched, stimulating group Ia afferent fibers ↓ Group Ia afferents synapse directly on α-motoneurons Stimulation of α-motoneurons leads to contraction of the muscle that was stretched to return it to its original length
What is its purpose?	To resist gravity; as muscle afterload increases, this reflex increases recruitment to stabilize the muscle group

Describe the Golgi tendon reflex:

Active muscle contraction stimulates group Ib afferent fibers in the Golgi tendon organs

↓

Group Ib afferents stimulate inhibitory interneurons in the spinal cord

↓   ↓

| α-Motoneurons inhibited, causing relaxation of the contracting muscle | Antagonistic muscles are activated |

What is the purpose of the Golgi tendon reflex?

To prevent muscle damage; if the force generated by the muscle risks injury to the muscle group, this reflex helps to modulate the output to prevent that injury

Describe the flexor withdrawal reflex:

Pain stimulates groups II, III, and IV flexor reflex afferent fibers

↓

Afferents synapse via interneurons to multiple motoneurons in the spinal cord

↓

Ipsilateral side: Flexors are stimulated to contract and extensors are inhibited, pulling the side away from the stimulus

Contralateral side: Flexors are inhibited and extensors are stimulated to maintain balance

What is the purpose of the flexor withdrawal reflex purpose?

To allow for rapid withdrawal of an appendage from a dangerous stimuli; the ipsilateral side contracts muscle groups to pull away, the contralateral side stabilizes the organism for that withdrawal

What is the persistent neural activity that is left in the polysynaptic circuit of the flexor withdrawal reflex called?

Afterdischarge

What is the function of the afterdischarge?

Prevents the muscle from relaxing for some time to maintain stability

What occurs with transection of the spinal cord below the lesion?

Loss of voluntary movement, conscious sedation, and reflexes (initially)

What occurs with time to the initial loss of reflexes with cord transection?

Partial return or may progress to hyperreflexia

A transection above what level will produce the following?

Loss of sympathetic tone to the heart   C7

Breathing cessation   C3

Death   C1

CORTICAL CONTROL OF MOTOR SYSTEMS

The execution of motor commands requires several layers of oversight. Where do the following occur?

Planning

The association cortex (planning) and the basal ganglia (goal-orientation)

Neural Output

The primary motor cortex, and the cerebellum

Execution

Spinal circuits (which include peripheral nerves)

What nerves are considered lower motor neurons?

Only those nerves whose cell bodies originate in the ventral gray matter

What are the pyramidal tracts?

Corticospinal tract and corticobulbar tract

Where do the corticospinal tracts originate and what are they carrying?

These primarily originate in the motor cortex and are carrying α-motoneurons

What are the extrapyramidal tracts and what is their purpose?

Lateral vestibulospinal tract: gross control of balance

Medullary reticulospinal tract: fine control of posture

Rubrospinal tract: redundant control for simple motor commands (walking)

Tectospinal tract: to direct the head and eyes toward a target (think of an owl and how it tracks prey $\rightarrow$ that is all tectospinal)

What are the functions of the cerebellum?	1. Influences rate, force, range, and direction of movement (spinocerebellum) 2. Plans and initiates movement (pontocerebellum) 3. Influences balance and eye movement (vestibulocerebellum)
What are the layers of the cerebellar cortex from outside in?	1. Molecular layer 2. Purkinje cell layer 3. Granular layer
What cell type is responsible for cerebellar output?	Purkinje cells
What type of output does the cerebellum produce?	Always inhibitory (read: corrective)
What is the neurotransmitter for the cerebellar output?	γ-Aminobutyric acid (GABA)
What is the function of the basal ganglia?	Plans and executes smooth movements by modulating thalamic outflow to the motor cortex
What are the components of the basal ganglia?	Striatum Globus pallidus Subthalamic nuclei Substantia nigra
How does the basal ganglia communicate with the thalamus and cerebral cortex?	Direct and indirect pathway
Which basal ganglia pathway has an overall inhibitory effect?	Indirect pathway
Which basal ganglia pathway has an overall excitatory effect?	Direct pathway
What is the neurotransmitter for communication between the striatum and substantia nigra?	Dopamine
Where is dopamine synthesized?	Substantia nigra
What effect does dopamine have on the following?	Dopamine tends to "lubricate the cogs" of the basal ganglia, encouraging cortical motor output
Direct pathway	Excitatory (D_1 receptors)
Indirect pathway	Inhibitory (D_2 receptors)

What is the effect of a lesion in the following locations?

    Striatum — Produces quick, continuous, "dance-like" movements (e.g., chorea)

    Globus pallidus — Produces inability to maintain postural support

    Subthalamic nuclei — Produces wild, flinging movements (e.g., hemiballismus)

    Substantia nigra — Produces cogwheel rigidity, tremor, and decreased voluntary movement

What disease produces signs similar to a lesion in the striatum? — Huntington disease

What disease produces signs similar to a lesion in the substantia nigra? — Parkinson disease

What are the functions of the premotor cortex and supplementary motor cortex? — Generate a plan for movement and transfer it to the primary motor cortex

Which cortex is utilized in *mental rehearsal* of a movement? — Supplementary motor cortex

What is the function of the primary motor cortex? — Execution of movement

What is the somatotopical organization of the primary motor cortex known as? — Motor homunculus

What occurs when epileptic events occur in the primary motor cortex? — Jacksonian seizure (Jacksonian march), which is a seizure that spreads through the primary motor cortex in succession and affects the corresponding muscle groups

What is the effect of lesions above the following locations?

    Lateral vestibular nucleus — Decerebrate rigidity

    Red nucleus — Decorticate posturing with intact tonic neck reflexes

    Pontine reticular formation (below the midbrain) — Decerebrate rigidity

Describe the posture of the following conditions:

Decerebrate rigidity

1. Arms are adducted and rigidly extended at the elbows
2. Forearms are pronated
3. Wrists and fingers are flexed
4. Feet are plantarflexed

Decorticate rigidity

1. Arms are adducted
2. Elbows, wrists, and fingers are flexed
3. Legs are internally rotated
4. Feet are plantarflexed

CEREBRAL CORTEX FUNCTIONS

What do electroencephalogram (EEG) potentials measure?

The sum of synaptic potentials in the pyramidal cells of the cerebral cortex across the cranium

What EEG waves predominate in the following conditions?

Alert and awake

Beta waves

Relaxing and awake

Alpha waves

Asleep

Slow waves

What is the function of the reticular activating system?

It determines arousal by projecting its output toward functions commanding executive function

What is the EEG rhythm that governs sleep called?

Circadian rhythm

Where is the day-night rhythm thought to be controlled?

Suprachiasmatic nucleus of the hypothalamus

What is the inherent operating cycle of the suprachiasmatic nuclei?

25 hours; it is modulated by nature's night-day cycle

What is REM sleep?

Rapid eye movement sleep

What does an EEG look like when someone is in REM sleep?

As if they were awake (e.g., beta waves predominate)

What occurs during REM sleep?

1. Eye movements
2. Pupillary constriction
3. Dreaming
4. Loss of muscle tone
5. Penile erection (in males)

How often does REM sleep normally occur?	Every 90 minutes
What happens to the duration of REM sleep with age?	It decreases
In what hemisphere is language dominant?	Left hemisphere
Does handedness affect the dominant language hemisphere?	No
What aspects of language are dominant in the right hemisphere?	Body language Facial expression Intonation Spatial tasks
Define aphasia:	Loss or impairment of the power to use or comprehend words
What type of aphasia are we dealing with when a person cannot understand written or spoken language?	Sensory aphasia
A lesion in what area will cause such an aphasia?	Wernicke area
What type of aphasia are we managing when a person can understand language, but not write or speak?	Motor aphasia
A lesion in what area will cause such an aphasia?	Broca area
How are short-term memories formed?	By changing synaptic connections
How are long-term memories formed?	By making structural changes in the nervous system (more stable)
Lesions to what will prevent formation of new long-term memories?	Bilateral lesions on the hippocampus
What allows for the transfer of information between the hemispheres of the cerebral cortex?	Corpus callosum

TEMPERATURE REGULATION

What structure regulates body temperature?

Anterior hypothalamus

How is body temperature regulated?

Core temperature is determined by temperature receptors on the skin and in the hypothalamus. This value is compared in the anterior hypothalamus with the set-point temperature. If the core temperature is off from the set-point, appropriate mechanisms are activated.

What are the body's heat-producing mechanisms and how do they work?

1. Shivering: posterior hypothalamus activates α- and γ-motoneurons causing muscle contraction and heat production
2. SNS: activates β receptors in brown fat to increase metabolic rate and produce heat (more effective in children)
3. Thyroid hormone: stimulates Na^+-K^+-ATPase to increase metabolic rate and produce heat

What are the body's mechanisms to get rid of excess heat and how do they work?

SNS: decreased tone to cutaneous blood vessels increases arteriovenous shunting of blood to venous plexuses close to the skin's surface and increases convection and radiation to produce heat loss (mediated by posterior hypothalamus)

Sweat glands: activated by sympathetic muscarinic receptors to produce heat loss by evaporation

What is a pyrogen?

Substance that increases the body's set-point temperature

How is fever mediated through a pyrogen?

Pyrogens increase interleukin-1 (IL-1) production
↓
IL-1 stimulates the anterior hypothalamus to produce prostaglandins
↓
Prostaglandins raise the set-point temperature

Define heat exhaustion:	Decreased blood pressure or syncope that develops from decreased blood volume due to excessive sweating
Define heat stroke:	Normal responses to increased ambient temperature are impaired and core temperature rises to the point of tissue damage
Define malignant hyperthermia:	Skeletal muscle produces excess heat through massive oxygen consumption and causes a rapid rise in body temperature
What commonly used agents can cause malignant hyperthermia?	Inhaled anesthetics
What agent is used to reverse malignant hyperthermia?	Dantrolene
Define hypothermia:	Normal responses to low ambient temperature are insufficient to maintain core temperature near the set-point

CLINICAL VIGNETTES

A 24-year-old chemistry major at a nearby university is brought to the emergency department (ED) after inadvertent exposure to hexamethonium.

What receptors are being influenced? Where are these found?

This is a ganglionic antagonist. It specifically blocks the neuronal nicotinic receptor (N_N). These are found in both the sympathetic and parasympathetic systems.

What are the clinical effects?

It leads to sympatheticolytic and parasympatholytic effects.

You, a neurologist, are asked to see a patient with some suspected sensory loss. You use two pins and slowly move the tips apart waiting for the patient to tell you when she feels two sharp points. On her hand, she tells you she can feel it when the tips are only a few millimeters apart, but on her back it takes several centimeters. You decide this is normal. What is the neurologic difference in these two regions?

Certain areas of the body (fingers, lips, etc) have sensory receptors with smaller receptive fields than others. This is called the two-point discrimination test.

A 27-year-old man was involved in a knife fight at a local bar. During that fight he suffered a knife wound to the back which has cleanly severed the right half spinal cord at the level of T7. What sensory deficits would he experience?

Think in terms of the ascending sensory tracts. Given that the right half has been severed, the dorsal column has yet to cross midline, whereas the anterolateral system has already crossed midline. As a result, he would have ipsilateral (same-sided) loss of proprioception and vibration sense, and contralateral (other-sided) loss of pain and temperature sensation.

Classically this is referred to as the Brown-Séquard syndrome, and is also characterized by spastic paralysis of ipsilateral muscle groups due to upper motor neuron destruction. Far more common than trauma, stroke can also cause this syndrome.

A patient with cystic fibrosis who has a long history of pancreatic dysfunction with steatorrhea comes to your office complaining of vision loss.

What do you suspect is going on?

Poor fat absorption tends to impair the absorption of fat-soluble vitamins (A, D, E, and K), the lack of vitamin A is the likely problem

Why is vitamin A important in the visual system?

It is activated to retinal which is imperative in rhodopsin function.

A 72-year-old man comes into your office complaining of hearing loss. A Weber test is performed and the sound lateralizes to the left ear.

What are the two possible deficits?

Conduction loss on the left, or sensorineural hearing loss on the right

If your Rinne test reveals air > bone bilaterally, but on the right the total air duration is only half what it is on the right, what is your diagnosis?

Sensorineural hearing loss on the right

What is most likely the underlying pathogenesis?

In a man of this age, this is most likely due to repeated exposure to loud noises with resultant destruction of hair cells

A researcher is performing experiments on the visual system in some test animals. What will be the effect on the animal's vision if transections in the following locations are made:

Single optic nerve

Ipsilateral blindness

Optic chiasm

Heteronymous bitemporal hemianopia

Optic tract

Homonymous contralateral hemianopia

Geniculocalcarine tract

Homonymous hemianopia with macular sparing

Drug X is an inhibitor of acetylcholinesterase (AChE) which has a very high affinity for acetylcholine (ACh). What would be the effect on the end-plate potential generated if drug X were given to someone?

Degradation of acetylcholine (ACh) would be blocked, so its accumulation in the motor synapse and its action would be prolonged and thereby producing a larger end-plate potential

A scientist is investigating a substance given to him by a colleague. He applies the substance to an autonomic ganglia and sees that action potential propagation is blocked. When he applies it to a neuromuscular junction, there is no change in action potential generation. What is the substance likely to be?

Hexamethonium, which is a nicotinic antagonist at the ganglion, but does not have an effect on the neuromuscular junction. It affects N_1 receptors, but not N_2 receptors.

A young woman met with an accident in which her left thalamic nucleus is destroyed. What is the physiologic consequence of this lesion?

She will have no sensation on the right side of her body

A previously healthy, 37-year-old man presents to his primary care physician (PCP) complaining of headaches that seem to be increasing in frequency. When further questioned, he notes that he has also been having blurry vision. A brain magnetic resonance imaging (MRI) reveals a 1.6 cm soft-tissue mass on the sella turcica with suprasellar extension. What structure has this tumor compressed to produce the visual symptoms?

The optic chiasm; classically, on examination, this will be presented as a narrowing of the visual field (bitemporal hemianopsia)

A 45-year-old man presents with new-onset vision deficit in the right eye. On examination, when the left eye is illuminated, both pupils constrict; while on illumination of the right eye, neither pupil changes. When the light is moved rapidly from the left eye to the right eye, the eyes constrict with exposure on the left and appear to dilate with exposure on the right. Where is the lesion?

The right retina or optic nerve

A 64-year-old woman complains of persistent nonproductive cough and weight loss of 7 to 10 lb in the past 3 months. On chest x-ray (CXR) and computed tomography (CT), a dense lesion in the right apex was visualized, which is later confirmed to be a carcinoma. On a subsequent follow-up visit, she reports deficiencies in her vision and you notice her face is not sweating, even in Arizona's 90°F weather. You notice that her right eyelid is drooping more so than previously. What do you suspect these symptoms mean?

The patient probably has a Pancoast tumor, which is compressing her sympathetic cervical ganglion causing Horner syndrome: miosis, ptosis, and anhydrosis.

A pugilist is struck in the nose and breaks his cribriform plate. After he recovers from his fight, he notices that his wife's perfume does not smell as strongly as it usually does. What is the likely mechanism for this change?

The broken cribriform has likely severed some of the input fibers to the olfactory bulb and produced hyposmia. A broken cribriform may also be heralded by CSF rhinorrhea.

A high school boy is fond of listening to rock music that favors heavy bass (low-frequency) tones. He also has a tendency to listen to music at very high volumes. Which part of the basilar membranes in his ear is at risk for serious damage?

The apices, which detect low frequencies

A young child accidentally touches a pot filled with boiling water. He quickly withdraws his hand from the pain, but simultaneously extends his other hand to maintain his balance. What caused the extension of the other hand?

Crossed extension reflex, which is part of the flexor withdrawal reflex and helps to maintain balance

A young female patient is in a car accident in which her spinal cord is injured. When she is rushed into the trauma bay, her legs are flaccid and reflexes cannot be obtained. The patient overhears these results and is very frightened. What do you tell her about the condition of her legs?

The patient is in spinal shock, whereby she has lost excitatory stimulation from both α- and γ-motoneurons. With time she may have partial recovery of muscle control and return of her reflexes with the possibility of hyperreflexia.

A 50-year-old man slipped while he was shoveling his driveway and hit his head. His wife brings him into the emergency room (ER). When the doctor goes to see him, it is noted that the man is unable to speak or write, but follows verbal commands. What type of injury has he suffered?

The man has a motor aphasia, which results from damage to Broca area

CHAPTER 3

Cardiovascular Physiology

ANATOMIC CONSIDERATIONS

How do arteries and veins differ in regard to the following?

	Arteries	Veins
Function	Deliver oxygenated blood to tissues	Return blood to the heart
Wall thickness	Thick-walled (due to elastic tissue and smooth muscle)	Thin-walled with valves
Pressures	High pressure	Low pressure

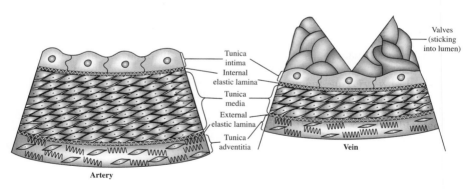

Figure 3.1 Arteries and veins: a structural comparison.

How does the heart receive its own blood flow?

The coronary arteries; they branch off in the first centimeter of the aorta

What is compliance?

Compliance describes the distensibility of a given structure

What is the formula for compliance? (Note: Compliance = Capacitance)

$$C = \frac{\Delta V}{\Delta P}$$

C = Compliance
V = Volume
P = Pressure

Which has a higher compliance, arteries or veins?

Veins

Which contains the larger proportion of blood, arteries or veins?

Veins contain a higher proportion of total blood volume; this is the unstressed volume, a reservoir that can be mobilized in times of need.

The wall of the aorta has one of the highest concentrations of elastin. What does this elastin do for circulation?

It facilitates the Windkessel effect; the heart pushes blood out into the low compliance aorta, which balloons slightly; subsequently, the elastin allows the aorta to force the blood forward into the systemic circulation

What is unique about the capillary bed of the vasculature? Why is that important?

It has the largest cross-sectional area and surface area, which allows for the efficient exchange of nutrients, water, and gases

What is unique about the pulmonary vasculature compared to the systemic vasculature?

Hypoxia causes vasoconstriction of the pulmonary vasculature. In most organs hypoxia causes vasodilation.

What is the effect of pulmonary hypoxic vasoconstriction?

It shunts blood toward lung segments that are being effectively ventilated

How does flow in the pulmonary circulation relate to flow in the systemic circulation?

They must be equal! While the total amount of blood in each circuit varies at any given time, total flow per unit time through each circuit must be equal.

HEMODYNAMICS

How do we calculate flow? Can we generalize that equation to the whole systemic circuit?

$$Q = \frac{\Delta P}{R_T}$$

Q = flow
P = change in pressure
R_T = total resistance

$$CO = \frac{(MAP - P_{RA})}{TPR}$$

CO = cardiac output
MAP = mean arterial pressure
P_{RA} = right atrial pressure
TPR = total peripheral resistance

How does increasing the pressure gradient influence flow through the circuit?

Increases the flow

What is Poiseuille equation for resistance?

$$R = \frac{8\eta l}{\pi r^4}$$

R = resistance
η = viscosity of blood
l = vessel length
r = vessel radius

What happens to the resistance if the radius of the blood vessel is reduced by 50%?

Increased by a factor of 16
($R \propto [1/r^4]$ so $1/[^1/_2]^4 = 16$)

How is resistance regulated physiologically?

Through the autonomic nervous system which modulates the tone of vascular smooth muscle to change vessel radius

Which component of the vascular system is the site of the highest resistance?

The arterioles; these have the greatest ability to change their radius, and, therefore, their resistance

What factors change the resistance of the vasculature system proportionally?

Viscosity and length of the vessel

What is the major determinant of viscosity in the vascular system?

The hematocrit is mostly responsible for the viscosity within the vascular system

In what pathologic states does viscosity increase?

Polycythemia
Hyperproteinemia
Hereditary spherocytosis

Poiseuille law gives us the resistance for a given vessel segment. What are the equations for summing the resistance of vascular segments in series? In parallel?

Series: $R_T = R_1 + R_2 + R_3 ...etc.$

Parallel: $R_T = \dfrac{1}{R_1} + \dfrac{1}{R_2} + \dfrac{1}{R_3} ...etc.$

R_T = total resistance
R_x = resistance of segment x

On which arterioles are α_1-adrenergic receptors found?

Skin
Renal circulation
Splanchnic circulation

On which arterioles are β_2-adrenergic receptors found?

Skeletal muscle

What is the significance of this variation in receptor expression?

By increasing resistance in nonessential circuits, we can shunt blood to vital systems during times of need (stress)

What is the equation for the velocity of blood flow?

$$v = \dfrac{Q}{A}$$

v = velocity of blood flow (cm/s)
Q = volume of blood flow (mL/s)
A = cross-sectional area (cm^2)

Why is velocity of blood flow in the aorta higher than that of the capillaries?

Velocity of blood flow is inversely proportional to cross-sectional area; the aorta has a relatively small cross-sectional area compared to that of the sum of all the capillaries

When is the systolic pressure measured?

At the peak of cardiac contraction

When is diastolic pressure measured?

At the nadir of cardiac relaxation

How can you calculate the pulse pressure?

Pulse pressure = systolic − diastolic

What is the major determinant of pulse pressure (PP)?

Stroke volume (SV), rising SV leads to a higher PP

What happens to the pulse pressure when the compliance decreases?

Increases (think: atherosclerosis)

What is the mean arterial pressure (MAP)?

Average arterial pressure with respect to time

How can you determine MAP?	$MAP = CO \times TPR$ or $MAP = \frac{1}{3}$ (systolic) + $\frac{2}{3}$ (diastolic) CO = cardiac output TPR = total peripheral resistance
Which is lower, venous pressure or right atrial pressure?	Atrial pressure; recall that pressure drives blood flow
What is meant by laminar flow?	The movement of fluid through vessels in an organized way (think: water in a garden hose)
What is turbulent flow?	Fluid movement that is disorganized (think: white water rapids)
What can we use to predict if flow will be laminar?	Reynolds number; it is useful as an index of turbulence
Physiologic variation in what parameter most influences the Reynolds number?	Viscosity (anemia reduces viscosity, polycythemia would increase it, etc)

ELECTROPHYSIOLOGY—CARDIAC ACTION POTENTIAL

What is cardiac excitability?	The ability of the cardiac muscle cells to conduct an action potential after being depolarized by an inward current
Conductance of what ion determines the resting membrane potential in cardiac muscle cells?	Like all other excitable cells, conductance to K^+
What is the resting membrane potential of nonpacemaker cardiac myocytes?	~90 mV, which is close to the K^+ equilibrium potential
What maintains the resting membrane potential?	Na^+-K^+-ATPase membrane protein
Again, what does it mean when a membrane *depolarizes*?	There is an inward current that brings positive charge into the cell
What does it mean when a membrane *hyperpolarizes* or *repolarizes*?	There is an outward current that removes positive charge from the cell

In the diagram of cardiac action potential below, label all of its phases and the currents that are responsible for them.

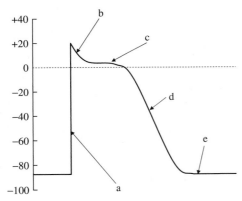

Figure 3.2   Cardiac action potential.

a) phase 0—inward Na^+
b) phase 1—inward Na^+ stops
c) phase 2—inward Ca^{2+}, some outward K^+
d) phase 3—max outward K^+
e) phase 4—Net ionic balance

Describe what happens during each of the following phases of a cardiac action potential:

Phase 0

Upstroke: caused by a rapid transient increase in Na^+ conductance, which allows an inward Na^+ current to depolarize the membrane (I_{Na})

Phase 1

Brief initial repolarization: caused by a decrease in inward Na^+ current due to closure of voltage-activated Na^+ channels

Phase 2

Plateau phase: caused by an increase in Ca^{2+} conductance and K^+ conductance continues to increase; this phase is marked by a net electrical balance between inward Ca^{2+} (I_{Ca}) and outward K^+ currents (I_{Kout})

Phase 3

Repolarization: K^+ conductance peaks. The Ca^{2+} conductance decreases; the electrical balance now favors the large outward K^+ current (I_{Kout})

Phase 4

Resting membrane potential: caused by an equilibrium between outward and inward ionic currents

All of these channels are triggered by what?

Threshold; the moment that threshold is reached, the sequence of cardiac conductance is set in motion.

What determines the peak of the cardiac action potential?

Conductance to Na⁺

ELECTROPHYSIOLOGY—ELECTROCARDIOGRAM

Identify the labeled parts and intervals of the electrocardiogram (ECG) below.

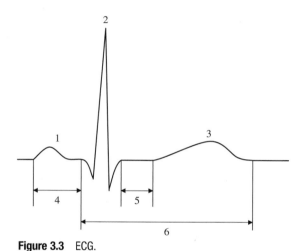

1. P wave
2. QRS complex
3. T wave
4. PR interval
5. ST segment
6. QT interval

Figure 3.3   ECG.

Define what the following waves/complexes from the ECG represent:

P wave

Atrial depolarization

PR interval

Conduction through the AV node

QRS complex

Conduction through the myocardium

QT interval

Mechanical contraction of the ventricle

T wave

Ventricular repolarization

How long does the PR interval last?

0.12 to 0.2 seconds (normally)

How long does the QRS complex last?

0.12 seconds (normally)

When does atrial repolarization occur?	During the QRS complex; it is not seen on the ECG because it is masked by the much greater electrical activity in the ventricle

What are the ECG changes associated with the following types of heart blocks?

1° (first degree)	PR interval > 0.20
2° (second degree) Mobitz type 1	PR intervals progressively increase from beat to beat until a beat is dropped
2° (second degree) Mobitz type 2	PR interval > 0.20 at a fixed interval with a fixed ratio of dropped beats
3° (third degree)	P waves (atrial contraction) and QRS complexes (ventricular contractions) are unrelated. Also called "complete heart block"

What are the ECG changes associated with the following abnormal rhythms?

Atrial fibrillation	No discernible P waves, irregularly spaced QRS complexes with an irregularly undulating baseline
Atrial flutter	"Sawtooth" baseline
Ventricular fibrillation	Completely abnormal rhythm that has no recognizable waves or complexes

ELECTROPHYSIOLOGY—PACEMAKER POTENTIAL

Where do pacemaker potentials occur normally?	1. Sinoatrial (SA) node 2. Atrioventricular (AV) node 3. His-Purkinje systems
What is the normal pacemaker of the heart?	The SA node
What is the normal pacing rate of the SA node?	60 to 100 potentials/min
What are the latent pacemakers in the heart?	AV node and His-Purkinje system

When might latent pacemakers take over for the main pacemaker?

Either when the SA node is suppressed or if conduction is blocked

What are the average pacing rates of the AV node and His-Purkinje system?

Average pacing rates are 45 and 30 beats/min, respectively

What is unique about the pacemaker action potential?

It has an unstable resting potential that exhibits slow phase 4 depolarization; this steady depolarization leads to repetitive cycles of action potential propagation

What phases are not present in the pacemaker potential?

Phases 1 and 2 are not present

On the cardiac pacemaker potential figure below, label all of its phases and the currents that are responsible for them.

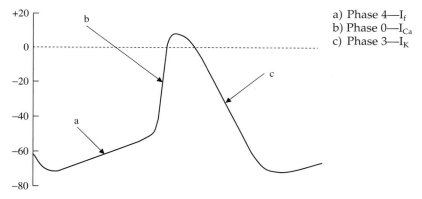

a) Phase 4—I_f
b) Phase 0—I_{Ca}
c) Phase 3—I_K

Figure 3.4 Cardiac pacemaker potential.

Describe what happens during each of the following phases of the pacemaker potential:

Phase 4

Slow depolarization: caused by a steady Na^+ conductance along with some Ca^{2+} conductance (I_f)

Phase 0

Upstroke: caused by an increase in Ca^{2+} conductance, which allows an inward Ca^{2+} current to depolarize the membrane toward the Ca^{2+} equilibrium potential (I_{Ca})

Phase 3

Repolarization: caused by an increase in K^+ conductance resulting in an outward K^+ current (I_K)

What is the name of the current that accounts for pacemaker activity?	Although it is predominately a Na^+ current, we call it I_f, the funny current
What turns on the current that accounts for the pacemaker activity?	Membrane repolarization leads to activation of I_f

ELECTROPHYSIOLOGY—CONDUCTION AND EXCITABILITY

What is conduction velocity?	The rate at which an electrical impulse propagates through cardiac tissue
Describe the anatomical flow of electrical propagation in the heart:	SA node generates an AP, this flows through the right atria (and to the left atria via Bachmann bundle) to the AV node. There it is delayed briefly before flowing through the His-Purkinje system into both ventricles concurrently.
What does conduction velocity depend on?	The magnitude of the inward current due to the influx of ions during phase 0 of the cardiac action potential
Where is conduction velocity the fastest?	Purkinje system
Where is conduction velocity the slowest?	AV node
What does the difference in conduction time between the AV node and the Purkinje system allow the heart to do?	The delay allows the ventricle to fill completely by accepting the "atrial kick"
What can happen if conduction velocity through the AV node is increased?	Ventricular filling can be compromised
What is a dromotropic effect?	A change in conduction velocity through a nerve fiber. When talking about the heart, we mean conduction through the AV node with changes in the PR interval
What type of dromotropic effect does the sympathetic nervous system produce?	Positive dromotropic effect (shortening of the PR interval)
Sympathetic stimulation of the heart utilizes what receptor? What is the neurotransmitter used?	β_1 receptor; norepinephrine (NE) is the neurotransmitter

How does the sympathetic nervous system produce its dromotropic effect?

By increasing the inward Ca^{2+} current during phase 4, this increase shortens the PR interval, thereby increasing the overall heart rate

What type of dromotropic effect does the parasympathetic nervous system produce?

Negative dromotropic effect (lengthening of the PR interval)

Parasympathetic stimulation of the heart utilizes what receptor? What is the neurotransmitter used?

Muscarinic receptor; acetylcholine (ACh) is the neurotransmitter

How does the parasympathetic system produce its dromotropic effect?

It decreases the inward Ca^{2+} current and increases the outward K^+ current; this decreased conduction velocity increases the PR interval, slowing the heart rate

How does dromotropy differ from chronotropy?

They are intimately related, but chronotropy refers specifically to *heart rate* as determined by the SA node; dromotropy more specifically refers to AV nodal conduction

Diagram and identify the following elements of a cardiac action potential.

Absolute refractory period (ARP)

Effective refractory period (ERP)

Relative refractory period (RRP)

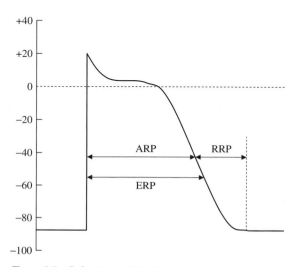

Figure 3.5   Refractory period relationships.

What is the ARP?	The time during which no number of entering impulses can initiate a new action potential
What is the ERP?	The time during which no conducted action potential can be produced
What is RRP?	The time during which an action potential can be initiated, but requires a larger depolarizing stimulus
What is the starting and ending point of the following refractory periods?	
ARP	Starts with the upstroke and ends after the plateau
ERP	Starts with the upstroke and ends slightly after the ARP
RRP	Starts right after the ARP and lasts until repolarization is complete

CARDIAC MUSCLE

In contrast to the neuromuscular junction of striated muscle, what is the stimulus for cardiac contraction?	Pacemaker potentials
What is a sarcomere?	Contractile unit of a myocardial cell
What is the role of the intercalated disk?	Maintains cell-to-cell cohesion and houses the gap junctions between cells
What is the role of the gap junction?	Provides a low-resistance path between cells, which allows for the rapid propagation of electrical impulses
What is the role of the T tubule?	Rapidly carries action potentials from the cell surface to the myocardial cell interior
What is the role of the sarcoplasmic reticulum (SR)?	Stores and releases Ca^{2+} for myocardial cell excitation-contraction coupling

What occurs in excitation-contraction coupling within the myocardium once the action potential enters the cell via the T tubules?

Ca^{2+} enters the cell from the extracellular fluid (ECF), creating an inward Ca^{2+} current
↓
Influx of Ca^{2+} causes the SR to release its stores of Ca^{2+}, further increasing the intracellular $[Ca^{2+}]$ (Calcium-induced calcium release)
↓
Ca^{2+} binds to troponin C molecules, which displaces the tropomyosin protein allowing the actin and myosin to bind, thereby generating contraction
↓
The SR reaccumulates the Ca^{2+}, which causes the myocardial cell to relax

What influences the amount of Ca^{2+} released by the SR during myocardial contraction?

Amount of Ca^{2+} stored in the SR and the size of the inward Ca^{2+} current

The magnitude of contraction for a myocardial cell is proportional to what variable?

The intracellular $[Ca^{2+}]$

Is reuptake of Ca^{2+} by the SR during relaxation of the myocardium an active or passive process?

It's an active process mediated by Ca^{2+}-ATPase pump

What is cardiac oxygen consumption related to?

It is directly related to the amount of tension developed in the cardiac muscle

What factors can increase cardiac oxygen consumption?

1. Increased afterload
2. Increased contractility
3. Increased heart rate (HR)
4. Hypertrophy of the cardiac muscle

(*Note*: All of these increase the amount of *work* that the cardiac muscle has to do.)

CARDIAC OUTPUT

What does the term "cardiac output" (CO) mean?

It is the total volume of blood pumped by the ventricle per minute

How can CO be expressed as a function of blood flow?

$$CO = \frac{(MAP - P_{RA})}{TPR}$$

MAP = mean arterial pressure
P_{RA} = right atrial pressure
TPR = total peripheral resistance

What is the expression for CO?

$$CO = SV \times HR$$

SV = stroke volume
HR = heart rate

CONTRACTILITY

What is contractility?

The ability of a muscle fiber to develop a force at a given muscle length

What is another term for contractility?

Inotropy

Can we alter the inotropic state of skeletal muscle?

No, it is a unique characteristic of cardiac muscle

What can be used as an estimate of contractility?

Ejection fraction (EF), which gives us a measure of how much blood is pushed out of the ventricle with each contraction

What is the expression for EF?

$$EF = \frac{SV}{EDV} \times 100\%$$

What is the normal range of EF?

The normal range of EF $\approx$ 55% to 80%

What is a positive (negative) inotropic agent?

Anything that causes an increase (decrease) in contractility

Generally speaking, what are some positive inotropes?

Sympathetic stimulation

Increased intracellular Ca^{2+}

Decreased extracellular Na^+

Cardiac glycosides

What are some negative inotropes?

Parasympathetic stimulation

β_1-blockade

Acidosis

Hypoxia

Hypercapnia

How does sympathetic stimulation increase contractility?

By increasing inward Ca^{2+} current during phase 2; G-proteins phosphorylate phospholamban proteins. This increases SR Ca^{2+} release providing more Ca^{2+} for excitation-contraction coupling.

What receptor does the sympathetic nervous system use to increase contractility?

β_1 receptors (Note: the same receptor used for dromotropic and chronotropic stimulation)

How does parasympathetic stimulation decrease contractility?

Muscarinic receptors are stimulated by ACh to decrease the inward Ca^{2+} current during phase 2 of cardiac depolarization

How do cardiac glycosides increase contractility?

Myocardial cell membrane Na^+-K^+-ATPase is inhibited, which diminishes the Na^+ gradient across the cell membrane. This increased intracellular $[Na^+]$ decreases Ca^{2+} efflux by the Na^+-Ca^{2+} exchange mechanism thereby increasing intracellular Ca^{2+}.

STARLING RELATIONSHIPS

What relationship is described by a Starling curve?

Change in SV that occurs due to changes in end-diastolic volume

What is the expression for SV?

$$SV = EDV - ESV$$
EDV = end-diastolic volume
ESV = end-systolic volume

The length-tension relationship refers to what idea?

That the length of the ventricular myocyte is proportional to the force of contraction the myocyte generates

What factors govern the Starling/ length-tension relationships?

1. Preload
2. Sarcomere length
3. Velocity of contraction at a fixed muscle length

Clinically, what is the equivalent to preload?

Ventricular EDV, which approximates the degree of myocyte stretch

What effect do venodilators have on preload?

They decrease it by allowing for pooling of venous blood, decreasing EDV

What are some things that can cause an increase in preload?

Increased blood volume

Sympathetic stimulation

Exercise (slight increase)

What is afterload equivalent to?

Diastolic arterial pressure

What is afterload proportional to?

Peripheral resistance

What effect do vasodilators have on afterload?

Decrease it

What happens to the Starling curve under the following conditions?

    Enhanced contractility

    Depressed contractility

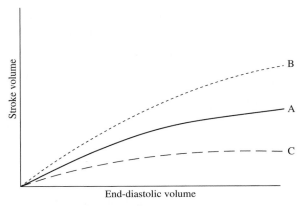

Figure 3.6   Frank-Starling curves.

In figure 3.6 above, what does the dashed line labeled "A" suggest?	It shows that as the end diastolic volume increases, so too does the total stroke volume.
In figure 3.6 above, what do the lines labeled "B" and "C" represent?	These show that with changes in cardiac inotropy, changes in end diastolic volume become more ("B") and less effective ("C"), respectively, at changing total stroke volume.
What can increase the contractility of the myocardium?	Pharmacologic stimulants Sympathetic stimulation Circulating catecholamines (epinephrine) Abrupt increase in afterload (Anrep effect) Increased HR (Bowditch effect)
What can decrease the contractility of the myocardium?	Pharmacologic depressants Parasympathetic stimulation Loss of myocardium Heart failure

CARDIAC CYCLE: PUTTING IT ALL TOGETHER

What are the steps of the cardiac cycle?

Ventricular diastole (passive filling)
↓ (a)
Atrial systole (active filling; "atrial kick")
↓ (b)
Isovolumetric ventricular contraction
↓(c)
Rapid ventricular ejection
↓ (d)
Reduced ventricular ejection
↓ (e)
Isovolumetric ventricular relaxation
↓ (f)
Repeat . . .

Use the letters next to the labeled arrows above to answer the following questions:

Closure of the mitral and tricuspid valves

(b) As the contracting myocardium pressurizes the ventricle, the atrioventricular valves shut.

Opening of the atrial and pulmonic valves

(c) When the ventricular pressure exceeds downstream vascular pressures, the valves open to allow for forward flow.

Closure of the atrial and pulmonic valves

(e) As the myocardium relaxes the pressure in the vascular beds will eventually prevent forward flow. To prevent reverse filling of the ventricles, these two valves slam shut.

Where systolic pressure is measured

(d) The peak of ventricular pressure is also the systolic blood pressure.

Opening of the mitral and tricuspid valves

(f) As the myocardium continues to relax, its pressure eventually falls below that of the atria and blood can begin filling the ventricles again.

Identify the labeled phases and events in the ventricular pressure-volume loop below.

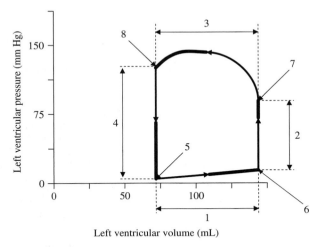

1. Ventricular filling "ventricular diastole"
2. Isovolumetric contraction
3. Ventricular ejection
4. Isovolumetric relaxation
5. Mitral valve opens
6. Mitral valve closes
7. Aortic valve opens
8. Aortic valve closes

Figure 3.7   Pressure-volume loop.

Describe what happens during the following phases of the cardiac cycle:

Isovolumetric contraction	Left ventricle (LV) begins filled with blood from the left atrium (LA). Upon excitation, the ventricle contracts and ventricular pressure increases, once LV pressure > LA pressure, the mitral valve closes. All valves are then closed and no blood is ejected, but the LV contraction continues and LV pressure increases.
Ventricular ejection	When LV pressure > aortic pressure, the aortic valve opens and blood is ejected out of the LV and into the aorta.
Isovolumetric relaxation	LV begins to relax and when LV pressure < aorta pressure, the aortic valve closes. All valves are closed at this point, but the ventricle continues to relax.
Ventricular filling	When LV pressure < LA pressure, the mitral valve opens and the ventricle begins to fill.

What is the volume of the ventricle before isovolumetric contraction?	End diastolic volume
What is the volume of the ventricle before isovolumetric relaxation?	End systolic volume

What happens to the pressure-volume loop under the following conditions and what causes these changes? Correlate these situations to the graphs on the following page.

    Increased preload

Increased preload results in an increase in EDV. This increase causes an increase in SV (due to Frank-Starling relationship), which is reflected as an increased width of the loop.

    Increased afterload

Increased afterload results from an increase in aortic pressure, which leads to a decrease in SV. This decreases the width of the loop.

    Increased contractility

Increased contractility leads to the ventricle developing greater tension during systole and increases the SV.

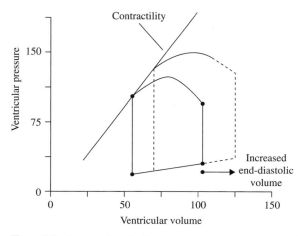

Figure 3.8 Increased preload curve.

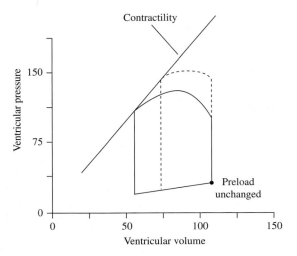

Figure 3.9   Increased afterload curve.

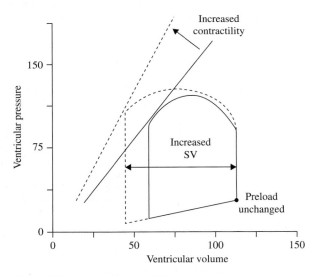

Figure 3.10   Increased contractility curve.

HEART SOUNDS AND MURMURS

What event does the first heart sound (S1) correspond to?	Mitral and tricuspid valve closure
What event does the second heart sound (S2) correspond to?	Aortic and pulmonic valve closure
What is a *split* S2?	When the aortic valve closes before the pulmonic valve
Is this split considered physiologic?	Yes, it can be. It is often called "the physiologic split."
What maneuver enhances the physiologic split?	Inspiration. The increased preload, leads to a delayed pulmonic closure, thereby widening the S2 split.
What are the potentially pathological heart sounds (gallops)?	S3 and S4
In what instances are the heart sounds not pathological?	S3: normal in children, and pregnant women S4: can be normal in kids and athletes, but standard mantra says "always pathologic"
Describe in words, the S3 and S4 heart sounds:	S3: immediately following isovolumetric relaxation, the mitral valve opens and blood rushes into a dilated ventricle; like water into a grocery bag S4: with atrial systole, the atria squeezes blood into a rigid ventricle (often secondary to hypertrophy), that rigidity is appreciated with the stethoscope as an S4
What pathology are the abnormal heart sounds associated with?	S3: dilated congestive heart failure (CHF) S4: hypertrophic ventricle
When would you hear the abnormal heart sounds?	S3: last third of diastole S4: just before S1 (during atrial systole)

Describe the murmurs associated with the following conditions. Also provide where they are best heard, and where they radiate to?

Aortic stenosis

Ejection click followed by a midsystolic crescendo-decrescendo murmur at second right interspace and radiates to carotids and apex

Aortic regurgitation

Blowing early diastolic murmur at the aorta and left sternal border, apical diastolic rumble (Austin Flint murmur), and midsystolic flow murmur at the base

Mitral stenosis

Opening snap followed by a delayed rumbling diastolic murmur at apex

Mitral regurgitation

Holosystolic high-pitched blowing apical murmur at the left sternal border

Mitral valve prolapse (MVP)

Late systolic murmur with midsystolic click

Ventricular septal defect (VSD)

Holosystolic murmur over entire precordium and heard maximally at the fourth left interspace

Patent ductus arteriosus (PDA)

Continuous machinelike murmur that is loudest at second left interspace

ARTERIAL PRESSURE REGULATION

What two physiologic systems are primarily responsible for BP management?

1. Baroreceptor reflex
2. Renin-angiotensin system

Through what reflex is the body able to quickly regulate the minute-to-minute arterial blood pressure?

Baroreceptor reflex

How is the baroreceptor reflex mediated?

It is a neurally mediated negative feedback system

What are baroreceptors?

Stretch receptors

Where are they located?

The primary receptors can be found at the bifurcation of the common carotids; another set is located in the aortic arch.

What do the baroreceptors respond to?	Carotid sinus baroreceptors: stretch of the sinus walls
	Aortic arch receptors: increases in aortic wall tension
What nerves do the baroreceptors utilize to regulate blood pressure?	Carotid sinus baroreceptors: glossopharyngeal nerve (CN IX)
	Aortic arch baroreceptors: vagus nerve
What is the primary difference between the two receptors?	Aortic arch baroreceptors primarily respond to *increases* in arterial pressures, carotid receptors are more sensitive to *decreases* in arterial pressures
What are the steps in the baroreceptor reflex?	The stretch receptors detect changes in vascular wall stretch. As pressure rises (or falls) the AP frequency in the afferent limb increases (or decreases).
	The autonomic response is coordinated by the vasomotor center and changes vascular tone to maintain normal blood pressure.

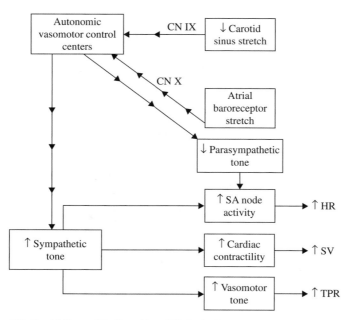

CN: Cranial Nerve, HR: Heart Rate, SV: Stroke Volume, TPR: Total Peripheral Resistance

Figure 3.11   Baroreceptor reflex.

What mediates the response of the vasomotor center?	Changes in parasympathetic and sympathetic tone
What autonomic responses does the vasomotor center utilize to maintain blood pressure?	Increased HR Increased contractility (with increased SV) Vasoconstriction of arterioles and veins
What happens during carotid massage?	Massage stretches the walls of the carotid artery, which is interpreted as an elevated BP
Where are the peripheral chemoreceptors located?	Carotid and aortic bodies
What do they respond to?	Decreased P_{O_2} Decreased pH of blood Increased P_{CO_2}
Where are the central chemoreceptors located?	Vasomotor center
Do the central chemoreceptors respond directly to P_{O_2}?	No
What do central chemoreceptors respond to?	Decreases in pH and increased P_{CO_2} of brain interstitial fluid (CSF)
What is the Cushing reaction?	Response to cerebral ischemia where increased intracranial pressure causes hypertension (sympathetic) and bradycardia (parasympathetic)
What is the body's long-term blood pressure regulation system?	Renin-angiotensin-aldosterone (RAA) system
How does the RAA system regulate blood pressure?	By adjusting total plasma volume
Describe how each of following are involved in the RAA system:	
Juxtaglomerular complex	Renal perfusion is measured by the juxtaglomerular apparatus (JGA) by sensing changes in afferent arteriolar wall tension; decreases in tension lead to increases renin secretion
Renin	Catalyzes the conversion of circulating angiotensinogen into angiotensin I
Angiotensin-converting enzyme (ACE)	Converts angiotensin I into angiotensin II

Where is ACE primarily located?	Lungs
What are the effects of angiotensin II?	1. Stimulates vasoconstriction of the arterioles, which increases TPR and MAP 2. Stimulates synthesis and secretion of aldosterone which causes an increase in Na^+ resorption and K^+ secretion in the distal tubule
What is the other name for antidiuretic hormone (ADH)?	Vasopressin
Where is ADH secreted?	Posterior pituitary
What causes the release of ADH?	Atrial baroreceptors detect changes in blood volume or blood pressure
What are the effects of ADH?	Increases TPR by causing peripheral vasoconstriction through V_1 receptors Increases water reabsorption by the renal distal tubule and collecting ducts with the activation of V_2 receptors
What causes the release of atrial natriuretic peptide (ANP)?	Increased atrial pressure due to higher venous returns
Where is ANP released?	The atria
What are the effects of ANP?	Increased Na^+ and H_2O excretion by the kidney to decrease blood volume and inhibits rennin, aldosterone, and ADH secretion

SPECIAL CIRCULATIONS

What percentage of cardiac output is directed to the following circulations?	
Brain	4%
Heart	15%
Kidneys	20%
Gut	25%

What is autoregulation?

Mechanism by which local vascular circuits are altered to meet the demands of specific tissues

What organs exhibit autoregulation?

Brain, heart, and kidney

What is active hyperemia?

Blood flow to the organ is proportional to the metabolic activity of the organ

What is reactive hyperemia?

Transient increase in blood flow to an organ after it has undergone a brief period of arterial occlusion (e.g., ischemia)

What mechanisms have been proposed to explain the local control of blood flow?

1. Myogenic hypothesis: based on vascular smooth muscle contracting when stretched and explains autoregulation, but not active or reactive hyperemia
2. Metabolic hypothesis: suggests that active tissue (or poorly perfused tissue) produces vasodilatory metabolites (e.g., CO_2, H^+, K^+, lactate, adenosine); this explains active and reactive hyperemia

What effects do each of the following have on the vasculature?

Histamine and bradykinin

Arteriolar dilation and venous constriction

5-hydroxytryptamine (5-HT, serotonin)

Arteriolar constriction

Prostacyclin and E-series prostaglandins (PGE_1 and E_2)

Vasodilation

F-series prostaglandins and thromboxane A_2

Vasoconstriction

What factors can influence autoregulatory set-points in the following locations?

Brain

Local metabolic factors: P_{CO_2}; a rising P_{CO_2} causes cerebral vasodilation

Heart

Local metabolic factors: hypoxia, adenosine, and nitrous oxide (NO)

Kidney

Myogenic and tubuloglomerular feedback

What factors determine autoregulation in skeletal muscle at rest and with exercise?	At rest: sympathetic innervation With exercise: local metabolic factors: lactate, adenosine, and K^+

MICROCIRCULATION AND LYMPHATICS

What is located at the junction between arterioles and capillaries?	Precapillary sphincter
Do capillaries contain smooth muscle?	No
What are capillaries composed of?	Single layer of endothelial cells and a surrounding basement membrane
As discussed above, what two features describes capillaries?	1. Low velocity flow 2. High surface area
How do small water-soluble substances enter capillaries?	Through pores (clefts) between adjacent endothelial cells
Can proteins fit through the pores?	Not normally, they are too large
Where are the pores the widest?	In the liver and intestine (sinusoids)
What is unique about the junctions in the sinusoids?	They are wide enough to allow the passage of proteins
How do large water-soluble substances enter capillaries?	Pinocytosis
How do lipid-soluble substances enter capillaries?	Through the membrane of the endothelial cells by simple diffusion
Where are the endothelial pores the tightest?	In the brain; their tight junctions help to create the blood-brain barrier
What are the components of the blood-brain barrier?	Endothelial cells of the cerebral capillaries and astrocytic foot processes
What substances pass readily through the barrier?	Lipid-soluble substances

What substances are excluded by the barrier?

Protein and cholesterol

What are the functions of the blood-brain barrier?

1. Maintains a constant environment for the neurons in the central nervous system (CNS)
2. Protects the brain from toxic substances
3. Prevents movement of neurotransmitter into the circulation

For the following compounds indicate where their concentration is higher, blood or cerebrospinal fluid (CSF)?

Ca^{2+}

Blood

Cholesterol

Blood (absent in CSF)

Cl^-

Equal in both

Creatinine

CSF

Glucose

Blood

HCO_3^-

Equal in both

K^+

Blood

Mg^{2+}

CSF

Na^+

Equal in both

Protein

Blood (absent CSF)

What equation governs fluid exchange across capillaries?

The Starling equation:

$$J_v = K_f ([P_c - P_i]) - ([\pi_c - \pi_i])$$

J_v = fluid movement (mL/min)
K_f = hydraulic conductance (mL/min · mm Hg)
P_c = capillary hydrostatic pressure (mm Hg)
P_i = interstitial hydrostatic pressure (mm Hg)
π_c = capillary oncotic pressure (mm Hg)
π_i = interstitial oncotic pressure (mm Hg)

Transcapillary fluid movement favors _____ **at the arteriolar end of the capillary and** _____ **at the venous end.**

Filtration, reabsorption

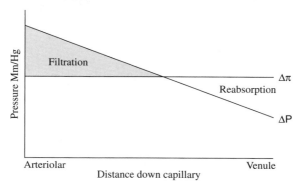

Figure 3.12   Starling forces in capillaries ΔP, hydrostatic pressure gradient; $\Delta \pi$, osmotic pressure gradient.

What can cause an increase in P_c?

Increased arterial or venous pressure

What can cause a decrease in π_c?

Decreased blood protein concentration

What can cause an increase in π_i?

Inadequate lymphatic function

What is lymph?

Excess fluid that is filtered out of capillaries and not reabsorbed

What is the function of the lymphatic system?

To collect and return excess fluid along with any filtered proteins back into circulation

What type of flow do the lymphatics demonstrate?

Unidirectional

What permits this type of flow?

One-way flap valves

What causes edema?

Essentially, most edematous states can be explained through variation in one of the Starling variables. This perversion results in more interstitial fluid than the lymphatics can return into the circulation.

CLINICAL VIGNETTES

A 36-year-old man suffers a gunshot wound to the upper thigh. After being rushed to the emergency department, the man is examined and it is found that he has a heart rate of 110, and a blood pressure of 86/40 and he seems cool and clammy to the touch.

What is happening?

He is losing blood volume into the soft tissues of the thigh.

How did the body detect this change?

The body is quickly able to detect blood volume changes through the baroreceptors of both the aortic arch and the carotids.

Why is his heart rate elevated?

To compensate for falling perfusion pressures, the body increases sympathetic output stimulating the heart to beat more rapidly.

A 56-year-old man suffers from the rupture of his abdominal aorta. He undergoes an emergent graft-based repair surgery during which the surgeon must clamp all arterial blood flow to the lower limbs for 90 minutes. The surgeon would like to remove the clamp, but he knows that when he does he must closely watch the patient's blood pressure. What two things are going on when the surgeon removes the clamp?

This is a classic question in the operating suite. Because the lower limbs have been deprived of O_2, the tissues have begun to use anaerobic metabolism to support themselves. With that there is a buildup of metabolic by-products (lactic acid, adenosine, cytokines etc), these are potent vasodilators.

When the clamp is removed the pressure will go down both because there is a new parallel large-volume vascular circuit added, and the release of these metabolic by-products into circulation leads to more vasodilation systemically.

A 57-year-old man comes in complaining of new onset chest pain. Twenty minutes later his descending abdominal aorta ruptures leading to massive blood loss. Sympathetic outflow leads to mobilization of what immediately available blood reserve?

The venous reserve; the unstressed volume can be quickly mobilized to compensate for acute hemorrhage. Remember: the arterial vessels carry only about 15% to 20% of total blood volume under normal resting state; the balance can be quickly recruited for use.

What happens to the stressed volume in older patients compared to younger ones?

It decreases since the capacitance of the arteries decreases with age.

A 72-year-old woman with known hypertension and diabetes is being examined by her primary care physician at a routine checkup when she mentions that every time she gets out of the shower, she feels very itchy all over. The physician is somewhat concerned and orders some laboratory work which lead him to diagnose her with polycythemia vera and her hematocrit is found to be almost twice what it was when he checked it 3 years earlier.

What hematologic variable has changed?

As the hematocrit rises, the viscosity of blood also rises

According to Poiseuille law, how will this influence her overall vascular resistance?

According to the equation: $R = \dfrac{8\eta l}{\pi r^4}$

As viscosity rises, so too will total resistance. Also worth noting that it will increase the Reynolds number and, therefore, increase the likelihood of turbulent flow.

An 8-year-old boy with no past medical history comes to your hospital because his mother has noticed that his face, hands and feet have become swollen over the past 3 or 4 days. She wasn't concerned at first, but it seems to be getting worse. Being an astute physician, you order just a urinalysis which reveals, as you suspected, that this boy is losing significant amounts of protein (albumin) in his urine.

What equation determines capillary fluid flux?

$$J_v = K_f \left([P_c - P_i] \right) - \left([\pi_c - \pi_i] \right)$$

In this boy, the loss of albumin leads to a reduction in the π_c value. As this falls, fluid extravasation increases, leading to the observed edema.

In this boy what is the most likely pathophysiology?

While, you may not know this yet, this is classical for minimal change disease, a glomerular disorder that allows for protein loss through the glomerular capillaries. For more info see Chap. 5.

A patient has a mean arterial pressure (MAP) of 70 mm Hg, a right atrial pressure (P_{RA}) of 10 mm Hg, and total peripheral resistance (TPR) is determined to be 10 mm Hg min/L. What is the cardiac output (CO)?

$$CO = \dfrac{(MAP - P_{RA})}{TPR}$$

Substituting in the numbers given:

$$CO = \dfrac{70 \text{ mm Hg} - 10 \text{ mm Hg}}{10 \text{ mm Hg min/L}} = 6 \text{L/min}$$

An elderly gentleman has bilateral carotid bruits that are audible with auscultation. What is the physiologic mechanism for the increased turbulence that creates this phenomenon?

As vessels narrow, the velocity of a blood flow through them increases. This increase in velocity increases the likelihood of turbulent flow

A 14-year-old boy is brought to the emergency room (ER) from his hockey game in which he was struck in the chest with the puck from a slap shot. He is unresponsive and a stat electrocardiogram (ECG) shows P waves and QRS complexes with no apparent association. What type of heart block is the patient in?

Third degree (3°) or complete heart block; in these cases, the atria are beating at their own pace, independently of the ventricles. There is no conduction through the AV node.

A 50-year-old woman comes in for a preoperative examination and has an ECG done that shows resting heart rate of only 50 bpm, with no P wave, a normal QRS complex, and a normal T wave. Where is the pacemaker of her heart located?

Atrioventricular (AV) node. It is important to note both the slowing of the pacemaker potentials and the loss of the P wave.

An electrician is working with a live wire when he is suddenly shocked. Just immediately preceding the shock his ventricles contracted. Why do they not contract again from the shock?

His ventricles are in the absolute refractory period, so no amount of electrical stimulation will trigger contraction.

A baby is born with a ventricular septal defect. What can be said about the blood flow out of the heart if the left ventricular pressure is greater than that of the right?

Pulmonary blood flow is greater than aortic blood flow from the left-to-right shunt that is present.

A patient is given an experimental drug, which the manufacturer claims to be a cardioselective ACh-analog. What type of effects will this drug have on the patient's heart rate and conduction velocities?

The drug will mimic parasympathetic stimulation and result in decreased heart rate, slower AV conduction, and increased PR interval

An innocent bystander is hit by a stray bullet in a drive-by shooting and begins to bleed profusely. What is the cardiac-directed autonomic response to the acute blood loss?

Increased sympathetic stimulation of his heart and vasculature and decreased parasympathetic stimulation of his heart

A 65-year-old man undergoes angioplasty of his left anterior descending coronary artery. After the procedure, the vessel's radius has doubled. What will be the change in resistance?

It will decrease by a factor of 16

*Remember: $R = \dfrac{8\eta l}{\pi r^4}$

A young woman who suffered severe total body burns is brought into the hospital with grossly edematous limbs. What is the physiologic cause for the edema?

Increased permeability of the capillaries to water (e.g., $\uparrow K_f$) from damage suffered by the burns

What is the direction of fluid movement and net driving pressure in a capillary where P_c is 32 mm Hg, P_i is 3 mm Hg, π_c is 26 mm Hg, and π_i is 3 mm Hg?

$$\text{Net pressure} = (P_c - P_i) - (\pi_c - \pi_i)$$
$$= (32) - (-3) - (26 - 3)$$
$$= +12 \text{ mm Hg}$$

Fluid will move out of the capillary since the net pressure is positive

A medical student is performing a cardiovascular examination on a 5-year-old patient and hears a third heart sound. What does an S_3 correspond to? Should he be concerned about this finding?

An S_3 corresponds to rapid relaxation of a ventricle during early diastole in response to cardiac filling. A third heart sound is considered normal in children, pregnant women, and athletes, but is pathological in most other individuals.

A middle-aged woman comes to the ER complaining of chest discomfort and a feeling of light-headedness. On examination, she has an irregularly irregular pulse. What abnormal rhythm is this patient likely experiencing?

Atrial fibrillation; whenever you hear "irregularly irregular," think: atrial fibrillation (A-fib)

A young man is stabbed in the chest during an altercation and begins to bleed into his pericardium. What happens to the cardiac output and pressure in his heart chambers from this situation?

Cardiac output: decreases

Pressure: equalizes in all four chambers

Remember your cardiac mechanics: As the blood moves into the pericardium, the amount of blood allowed into the heart falls; as the condition worsens, the pressures across the valves and between chambers equalize and impairs the forward flow of blood through the heart

CHAPTER 4

Respiratory Physiology

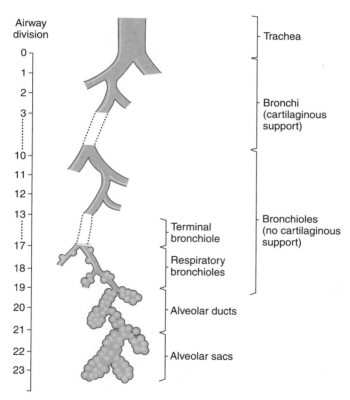

Airway division

0
1
2
3
⋮
10
11
12
13
⋮
17
18
19
20
21
22
23

Trachea

Bronchi (cartilaginous support)

Bronchioles (no cartilaginous support)

Terminal bronchiole

Respiratory bronchioles

Alveolar ducts

Alveolar sacs

Figure 4.1 Branches of the respiratory tree. (Reproduced, with permission, from Kibble JD, Halsey CR: *Medical Physiology: The Big Picture.* New York, NY: McGraw-Hill; 2009.)

RESPIRATORY ANATOMY

What is the purpose of the branching pattern shown above?	To allow for dramatic increase in cross-sectional area.
What is the approximate cross-sectional area of the trachea?	2.5 cm^2
How many alveoli are there present in a normal adult?	About 300 million
How many branches are there in the respiratory tree?	23
How many generations until alveoli are present; that is, how many branch generations in the conducting zone?	16 (trachea to the terminal bronchioles)
What type of epithelium lines the conducting zone?	Ciliated, pseudostratified columnar (also known as respiratory epithelium)
At what point in the respiratory tree does gas exchange begin?	Respiratory bronchioles (branch point 17)
What is the surface area of alveolar-capillary interface available for gas exchange?	50 to 100 m^2; approximately the size of a tennis court
What are the barriers to gas exchange at the alveolar-capillary interface?	Surfactant Alveolar epithelium Interstitial space Capillary endothelium
What types of cells compose the alveolar surface?	Type I pneumocytes: thin cells that constitute 90% of the surface area, even though less abundant than type II cells in numbers Type II pneumocytes: most abundant, but only constitute 10% of surface, and produce surfactant Phagocytic alveolar macrophages: ingests and clears foreign, inhaled particles
What are the two types of dead space?	1. Anatomic dead space (respiratory tree with no alveoli present) 2. Alveolar dead space (alveoli with no perfusion)

How is anatomic dead space approximated?

Ideal body weight in pounds is roughly equivalent to anatomic dead space in milliliters.

What is the function of anatomic dead space?

Warm and humidity inspired air

Removal of foreign particles

In which locations and by what mechanisms is air filtered?

1. In vibrissae (aka nasal hairs)
2. By mucus in bronchi and bronchioles
3. Alveolar macrophages remove particles that make it to alveoli

What is the mucociliary escalator?

As foreign particles are trapped in the mucus that lines the epithelium of the respiratory tract, the cilia on the epithelium beat upwards, away from alveoli and lower respiratory structures.

What common inhalant inhibits the mucociliary escalator?

Cigarette smoke

Why do particles in venous blood not reach the arterial circulation?

They are filtered out by the pulmonary circulation (these particles can vary, but can be clots, agglutinated red blood cells, gas bubbles, etc).

What does this "filter" prevent?

Thrombotic or occlusive events on the left side of circulation (such as stroke, MI, etc)

LUNG VOLUMES AND CAPACITIES

Define the following lung volumes:

Tidal volume (V_T)

Volume of a normal breath at rest (average 500 mL)

Inspiratory reserve volume (IRV)

Additional volume of gas that can be inspired above the V_T (average 3 L)

Expiratory reserve volume (ERV)

Volume of gas that can be forcefully expired after a normal passive expiration (average 1.3 L)

Residual volume (RV)

Volume of gas that remains after maximal expiration (average 1.5 L)

| How are lung volumes and capacities related? | A capacity is the sum of two or more volumes |

Define the following lung capacities:

Total lung capacity (TLC)	Volume of gas present after a maximal inspiration (average 6 L)
Vital capacity (VC)	Maximal volume that can be expelled after a maximal inspiration (average 4.5 L). This is the maximal volume that can be exchanged in a single breath
Functional residual capacity (FRC)	Volume remaining at the end of a normal breath at rest (average 3 L)

Identify the labeled lung volumes on the spirogram below.

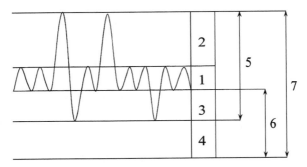

Figure 4.2 Lung volumes.

1. Tidal volume (V_T)
2. Inspiratory reserve volume (IRV)
3. Expiratory reserve volume (ERV)
4. Residual volume (RV)
5. Vital capacity (VC)
6. Functional reserve capacity (FRC)
7. Total lung capacity (TLC)

What are the volumes that make up the following capacities?

Inspiratory capacity (IC)	$IC = V_T + IRV$
FRC	$FRC = RV + ERV$
VC	$VC = ERV + V_T + IRV$
TLC	$TLC = RV + ERV + V_T + IRV$

| Which lung volumes and capacities cannot be measured using spirometry? | RV, FRC, and TLC |

How can the above capacities be measured?	Nitrogen washout Helium dilution Body plethysmography
How does FRC change with position?	FRC increases when standing/sitting and decreases when supine
How does age affect the following parameters of pulmonary function tests (PFTs)?	
TLC	Decreased
RV	Increased
VC	Decreased
FRC	Does not change
Define minute ventilation (V_E):	Volume of air inspired or expired per minute: $$V_E = V_T \times \text{frequency}$$
What are:	
Forced vital capacity (FVC)	Volume exhaled with maximal expiratory effort
Forced expiratory volume in 1 second (FEV$_1$)	Volume that can be forcefully expired in 1 second
What is the normal ratio of FEV$_1$ per FVC?	80% (FEV$_1$/FVC = 0.8)
What is alveolar ventilation?	The volume of air reaching the alveoli per minute
Why is alveolar ventilation less than minute ventilation?	Last part of inspired air only reaches the conducting zone and never reaches the respiratory zone
How does shallow versus deep breathing affect alveolar ventilation?	Rapid shallow breathing produces much less alveolar ventilation; most of each breath ventilates the conducting zone
How is dead space calculated?	$$V_d = V_t \times ([Pa_{CO_2} \times Pe_{CO_2}]/Pa_{CO_2})$$ V_d: Dead space volume V_t: Total lung volume Pa_{CO_2}: Partial pressure of arterial CO_2 Pe_{CO_2}: Partial pressure of expired CO_2

RESPIRATORY MECHANICS

What are the muscles of inspiration?

1. Diaphragm (majority of work at rest)
2. External intercostals (increase thoracic size and prevent retraction)
3. Accessory muscles of inspiration (not used during quiet breathing)

What are the accessory muscles of inspiration?

Sternocleidomastoid, scalenes, strap muscles of neck

What is the innervation of the diaphragm?

Phrenic nerve (C3,4,5 keep the diaphragm alive)

Where does referred diaphragmatic pain occur?

Ipsilateral shoulder (remember the dermatomes of the nerve roots!)

Does the diaphragm contribute more to inspiration while supine or standing?

Supine; when standing, external intercostals contribute significantly

What action does the diaphragm perform?

As it contracts it flattens into the abdominal cavity, increasing the volume of the thoracic cavity

Which muscles are involved in normal, quiet expiration?

None. It is a passive process due to the elastic recoil by the lungs.

Which muscles are active in active expiration (e.g., exercise)?

Abdominal muscles and internal intercostals

During quiet breathing, which is longer, inspiration or expiration?

Expiration, in about a 2:1 ratio

Where is the intrapleural space?

It is between the lung and the chest wall. It is actually only a "potential space" under normal conditions because the visceral and parietal pleural layers are usually closely apposed.

What is the normal intrapleural pressure at rest?

Slightly subatmospheric (−3 to −5 cm H_2O)

How can the intrapleural pressure be measured?

A swallowed balloon can measure the intrathoracic pressure, which approximates the intrapleural pressure.

What is the normal series of events during inspiration?

Respiration initiated by central nervous system
↓
Diaphragm contracts, along with other external intercostals
↓
Thoracic volume increases
↓
Decrease in intrapleural pressure
↓
Alveoli expand
↓
Alveolar pressure becomes subatmospheric
↓
Air flows into alveoli to equilibrate with atmospheric pressure

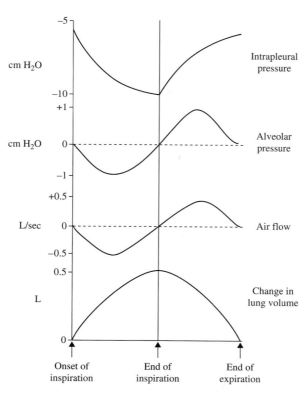

Figure 4.3 Volume, pressure, and airflow during a respiratory cycle.

Define compliance (C):

An indication of how easily the lungs and chest wall can be stretched or inflated. In general terms, it refers to the lungs ability to accommodate incoming volume.

What is the equation for compliance?

$$C = \Delta V / \Delta P$$
ΔV = change in volume
ΔP = change in pressure

What physiologic elements influence compliance?

Most widely discussed are things like intrinsic recoil of pulmonary tissues, but remember that lung volume and alveolar surface tension also contribute

What processes can cause a decrease in compliance?

Pulmonary congestion and various restrictive lung diseases

What causes an increase in compliance?

Destruction of lung tissue with concomitant loss of elastic tissues (e.g., emphysema)

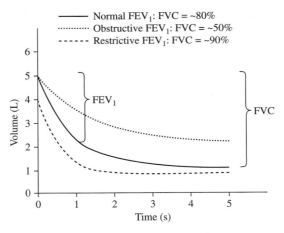

Figure 4.4 Comparison of spirograms between normal and diseased lungs.

Compare the FEV_1: FVC ratio of a normal lung to a lung with emphysema or chronic bronchitis (COPD)

Normal lung has an FEV_1: FVC ratio of 80%, emphysematous lung has an FEV_1: FVC ratio of <80% (usually 60%-70% or less).

What other obstructive lung disease cause this pattern?

Asthma, bronchiectasis

What physical examination findings correlate with obstructive lung disease?

Increased anteroposterior diameter of the chest (barrel chested), and prolonged expiratory phase

How does the FVC compare between a normal lung and one with restrictive disease?

Total FVC is lower due to decreased lung compliance

How does compliance change with lung volumes?

Increases at low volumes, decreases at high volumes

Define elasticity:

The recoil force generated by distension of a structure

How is compliance related to elasticity?

Inversely ($C = 1/E$)

What contributes to the lungs' recoil properties?

Lung parenchyma (elastin, collagen, etc)

Surface tension at air-liquid interface in alveoli

How does Laplace law relate to surface tension, and how does that affect the collapsibility of alveoli?

$$P = \frac{2T}{r}$$

P = collapsing pressure (dyne/cm^2)
T = surface tension (dyne/cm)
r = alveolar radius (cm)

Which is easier to keep open, a large alveoli or a small one?

Large alveoli (alveolar radius is inversely proportional to collapsing pressure, see above equation)

Which cells produce surfactant?

Type II alveolar epithelial cells

What are the functions of pulmonary surfactant?

1. Reduce surface tension at low lung volumes (prevent atelectasis)
2. Increase surface tension at high lung volumes (contribute to lung recoil)
3. Increase alveolar radius
4. Reduce pulmonary capillary infiltration

What is the effect of surfactant on compliance and elasticity?

Surfactant increases compliance, and decreases elasticity

What is surfactant composed of?

1. Dipalmitoyl phosphatidylcholine (aka lecithin)-major
2. Phosphatidylglycerol
3. Other lipids
4. Neutral lipids
5. Proteins

How may surfactant synthesis be reduced?

Developmental deficiency (e.g., prematurity)

Hypovolemia

Hypothermia

Acidosis

Hypoxemia

Rare genetic disorders of surfactant synthesis

What is the significance of surfactant in infant respiratory distress syndrome (IRDS)?

In this condition a surfactant deficiency results in high surface tension in the alveoli of the lungs, leading to alveolar collapse and atelectasis. Because of this, there is decreased FRC with subsequent arterial hypoxemia.

What does the therapy for IRDS include?

1. Positive end-expiratory pressure (PEEP)
2. Steroids
3. Exogenous surfactant

By what week do the fetal lungs make surfactant?

Week 34 to 36

What may indicate fetal pulmonary maturity?

The ratio of lecithin to sphingomyelin or L/S ratio in the amniotic fluid. Over the course of gestation, lecithin gradually increases with pulmonary maturity while the sphingomyelin remains constant, so it serves as a useful meter.

The presence of minor phospholipids (e.g., phosphatidylglycerol) is also indicative in cases where the L/S ratio is borderline.

What L/S ratio usually indicates pulmonary maturity?

2:1

What can be used to help accelerate the maturation of surfactant in the lungs of a fetus?

Glucocorticoid hormones

Under normal conditions, what structural feature of individual alveoli helps to prevent them from collapsing?

Alveolar walls and airway walls are structurally connected so that tension on alveolar walls created by one collapsing alveolus helps to hold adjacent alveoli open.

What is the above theory called?	Alveolar interdependence
What two types of resistance make up pulmonary resistance?	1. Airway resistance (~80%) 2. Pulmonary tissue resistance (~20%)
In what pathologic states is pulmonary tissue resistance increased?	Fibrosis from any cause, examples include amyloidosis and sarcoidosis
What factors determine airway resistance?	Gas viscosity Diameter of the airway Length of the airway
What law describes airway resistance?	Poiseuille law:

$$R = \frac{8\eta l}{\pi r^4}$$

R = resistance

η = viscosity of inspired gas

l = length of airway

r = radius of airway

How are airway resistance and airflow related?	Much like flow through the cardiovascular system, they are inversely related:

$$Q = \frac{\Delta P}{R}$$

Q = airflow (L/min)

ΔP = pressure gradient (cm H_2O)

R = airway resistance (cm/H_2O/L/min)

Which part of the respiratory system is the major site of airway resistance?	Medium-sized bronchi
Which part of the respiratory system has the highest individual resistance?	Small terminal airways; they are not the major site of airway resistance because they are far more numerous and are arranged in parallel
What factors can change airway resistance?	Altering the radius of the airways Changes in lung volume Viscosity/density of the inspired gas
What is bronchoconstriction/dilation?	Changes in the diameter of conducting airways

What causes bronchoconstriction?	Parasympathetic discharge
	Substance P
	Adenosine
	Hypersensitivity response (e.g., histamines)
	Arachidonic acid metabolites (e.g., prostaglandins and leukotrienes)
How does bronchoconstriction affect airways?	1. Reduces airway radius 2. Increases resistance 3. Via the above two changes, limits airflow during inspiration or expiration
What causes bronchodilation?	Sympathetic discharge and sympathetic agonists via β_2 receptors
How do obstructive diseases affect respiratory mechanics?	Increase airway resistance; it creates air trapping which increases lung volumes
How do restrictive diseases affect respiratory mechanics?	Decrease compliance, affecting inspiration mechanics; more on this later

GAS EXCHANGE

How are partial pressures determined?	Dalton law:
	$$P_P = P_T \times \text{fractional (gas)}$$
	P_P = partial pressure P_T = total pressure fractional [gas] = gas concentration
What is the fraction of oxygen in ambient air?	21%
What is the fraction of carbon dioxide in ambient air?	0.04% (can assume atmospheric CO_2 is equal to zero)

What are the partial pressures of O_2 and CO_2 in the following locations?

Atmospheric air	O_2: 160 mm Hg, CO_2: 0 mm Hg
Air in the trachea	O_2: 150 mm Hg, CO_2: 0 mm Hg
Alveolar air	O_2: 100 mm Hg, CO_2: 40 mm Hg
Arterial blood	O_2: slightly < 100 mm Hg, CO_2: 40 mm Hg
Mixed venous blood	O_2: 40 mm Hg, CO_2: 46 mm Hg

Why is the P_{O_2} in the trachea less than that of the atmosphere?

The air in the trachea is humidified (addition of H_2O, which decreases P_{O_2})

Why is the P_{O_2} in arterial blood slightly less than 100 mm Hg?

Regional V/Q mismatching and normal physiologic shunt

What is a *physiologic shunt*?

The ~2% of systemic cardiac output that bypasses the pulmonary circulation (bronchial circulation)

True or false? The composition of alveolar gas remains relatively constant at rest.

True

Why does alveolar gas composition remain constant at rest?

Because the FRC (2.8 L on average) is much larger than the tidal volume (0.5 L on average), creating a steady state environment for P_AO_2 and P_ACO_2

Define gas exchange:

Transport of gas from alveoli to hemoglobin (Hb) in the blood across the respiratory membrane

Where in the respiratory system does gas exchange occur?

In the terminal portions of the airways (respiratory bronchioles, alveolar ducts, and alveoli)

At rest, how long does it take for the blood to traverse the pulmonary capillaries?

It takes only 0.75 second for blood to move through the portion of the capillary where gas exchange occurs

What happens to this time during exercise?

Decreases (down to 0.25 seconds under strenuous exercise)

What factors determine pulmonary gas diffusion?

1. Surface area for diffusion
2. Partial pressure difference across membrane
3. Thickness of barrier
4. Diffusivity of gas

What equation governs pulmonary gas diffusion?
(Note: Don't commit this to memory.)

Fick equation:

$$V_{gas} \propto \left(\frac{A}{Th}\right) \times D \times (P_C - P_A)$$

V_{gas} = flow of gas across an area
A = area of barrier
Th = thickness of barrier
D = diffusion coefficient
P_C = partial pressure of gas in the pulmonary capillary
P_A = partial pressure of gas in the alveoli

Define the diffusion coefficient:
(Note: Don't commit this to memory.)

$$D \propto \frac{Sol_{gas}}{\sqrt{MWt}}$$

D = diffusivity factor
Sol_{gas} = gas solubility in tissue fluid
MWt = molecular weight

Explain flow limitation:

Gases enter the blood more quickly than the blood transverses the pulmonary capillaries. Therefore, the limiting factor in the amount of gas into the blood is not the diffusion through the membrane but the flow of blood through the capillaries.

What is another name for flow limitation?

Perfusion limitation

How can flow limitation be overcome?

By increasing blood flow (e.g., increasing cardiac output during exercise)

Which gases are subject to flow limitation?

N_2O, O_2

Explain diffusion limitation:

Gases diffuse into the blood more slowly than blood flows through pulmonary capillaries. Therefore, the limiting factor is the rate of diffusion into the blood, not the amount of blood flowing through the capillaries.

What is an example of a gas that is subject to diffusion limitation?

Carbon monoxide (quickly binds hemoglobin, but does not dissolve well in blood)

What is the significance of diffusing capacity (D_L)?

Its measurement permits evaluation of the diffusion properties of alveolar-capillary membrane by measuring the rate of gas transfer (conductance) by the respiratory system

Can oxygen be subject to diffusion limitation?

Yes. In pathologic states.

GAS TRANSPORT

How is O_2 transported in blood?

In arterial blood at P_{O_2} 100 mm Hg, P_{CO_2} 40 mm Hg, and Hb 97% saturated

Major: chemical combination with Hb (19.5 mL O_2/100 mL blood)

Minor: dissolved in the plasma (0.29 mL O_2/100 mL blood)

What is the partial pressure (oxygen tension) of normal O_2 arterial blood?

85 to 100 mm Hg

In normal adults, what are hemoglobin molecules (HbA) composed of?

Two α and two β chains. There are exceptions: fetal hemoglobin and disease states

What are the functions of hemoglobin?

1. Facilitates O_2 transport
2. Facilitates CO_2 transport
3. Buffers pH of the blood
4. Facilitates NO transport

What is heme?

Complex made up of a porphyrin ring and one atom of ferrous iron (there is one heme group per chain)

What is the role of the ferrous iron (Fe^{2+})?

Each ferrous iron reversibly binds one O_2 molecule making four binding sites per hemoglobin molecule

What is the significance of the iron in heme?

It has six available orbitals for binding, four to the pyrole groups of the porphyrin ring, one to the polypeptide chain, and one that can associate with oxygen

How does the hemoglobin structure affect its oxygen-carrying capacity?

Hemoglobin has a quaternary structure that varies in its affinity for oxygen depending on the number of oxygen bound to it.

How are the hemoglobin subunits affected in a deoxygenated state?	Hemoglobin subunits are in a *tense (tight)* configuration with a relatively lower affinity for O_2
How are the hemoglobin subunits affected when they have oxygen attached to them?	With each progressive O_2 molecule, hemoglobin takes on a *relaxed* configuration where subsequent binding of O_2 is facilitated as each O_2-binding site is exposed (called allosterism)
How does Hb affect the O_2 content in blood?	Increases the amount of O_2 that can be carried in the blood almost 70-fold
What percent of O_2 in arterial blood is carried by hemoglobin?	~98.5%
Define hemoglobin saturation:	Percent of hemoglobin that is combined with O_2
What influences the amount of O_2 that combines with hemoglobin?	O_2 tension (P_{O_2}) or O_2 saturation
Define O_2 capacity:	The maximal amount of O_2 that can be carried in the blood by hemoglobin
What is the hemoglobin-oxygen dissociation curve?	The curve relating percent saturation of the O_2-carrying capacity of hemoglobin to the P_{O_2} (see Fig. 4.5)
How does the sigmoid curve affect oxygen delivery at the:	
Plateau	Complete saturation can be ensured across many P_{O_2} values.
Steep section	Small change in P_{O_2} results in large changes in O_2 saturation. This facilitates unloading of oxygen at tissues.
Where in the human body are the following parts of the sigmoid curve most important?	
Plateau	Pulmonary capillaries
Steep section	Tissue capillaries
What does decreased oxygen affinity mean?	A higher P_{O_2} is required for hemoglobin to bind a given amount of O_2.

What factors decrease the affinity of hemoglobin for oxygen?

In general, think of exercise and altitude
1. Low pH (acidosis—increased H^+)
2. Increased P_{CO_2}
3. Increased temperature
4. Increased 2,3-diphosphoglycerate (2,3-DPG) concentration

What factors cause an increase in 2, 3-DPG concentrations?

1. High pH
2. Thyroid hormone
3. Growth hormone
4. Androgens
5. High altitudes

What is meant by a "left shift"?

As the Hb dissociation curve shifts to the left, it saturates *at a lower* P_{O_2}, but is more reluctant to unload O_2.

As an example, think of fetal Hb. It has a higher affinity for O_2 (a "left shift"), so it will "steal" O_2 from maternal Hb, but it is less eager to unload O_2 in the fetal tissues.

What is the P_{50}?

It is the P_{O_2} where the Hb is 50% saturated with oxygen. It is a useful measure of Hb kinetics.

Diagram the Hb dissociation curve and then diagram both a left and right shift of the curve noting how the P_{50} changes.

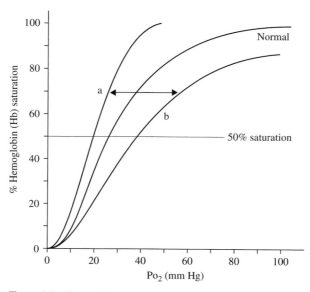

Figure 4.5 Hemoglobin saturation curve.

What does decreased oxygen affinity favor?	Oxygen delivery to tissue
In the above diagram, does the line labeled "b" have a higher or lower P_{50}?	Higher
How does that new P_{50} value relate to O_2 affinity/unloading?	That line represents decreased affinity/ increased oxygen unloading. The opposite is true for the line labeled "a."
What is the Bohr effect?	Decreased Hb affinity for oxygen due to lowered pH. This is related to the fact that protonated Hb (HbH) binds oxygen less avidly.
Where is the Bohr effect used physiologically?	In the peripheral tissue (helps unload oxygen in metabolically active tissues)
In Fig. 4.5, which curve represents the Bohr effect?	The curve that has shifted to the right (b)
How does fetal hemoglobin (HbF) differ from adult hemoglobin (HbA)?	HbF contains γ-polypeptide chains instead of β chains
What is the significance of the γ chains versus the β-chains HbF?	There is poor binding of 2, 3-DPG by the γ chains causing HbF to have greater affinity for O_2 than HbA.
How does anemia affect 2,3-DPG concentration in red blood cells (RBCs)?	Increases it
How is myoglobin in muscle different from hemoglobin in blood?	Myoglobin binds one, rather than four, molecules of O_2 per protein. This results in a rectangular hyperbolar dissociation curve, typical of Michaelis-Menten kinetics.
How does the dissociation curve of myoglobin affects its O_2 uptake relative to hemoglobin?	The myoglobin curve lies to the left of the hemoglobin curve indicating a greater O_2 affinity. It steals O_2 from hemoglobin and releases O_2 only at low Po_2 seen in tissues.
Where is much of the myoglobin found?	In skeletal muscles
What does decreased arterial O_2 content cause?	Decreased hemoglobin saturation and reduced arterial O_2 tension
For which does Hb have more affinity, CO or O_2?	CO (~200 × greater affinity)

What is formed as a result of CO reacting with hemoglobin?

Carboxyhemoglobin

How does carboxyhemoglobin formation affect O_2 content?

Decreases the functional Hb concentration

Reduces oxygen-carrying capacity of blood

Lowers the tissue O_2 tension

How is CO_2 transported in blood?

1. As HCO_3^- in plasma (major)
2. Dissolved in plasma or in RBCs (minor)
3. Formation of carbamino-Hb in RBCs (minor)
4. Formation of carbamino compounds with plasma protein (minor)

Where does hydration of CO_2 into HCO_3^- occur?

RBCs

What enzyme catalyzes the conversion of CO_2 into HCO_3^-?

Carbonic anhydrase catalyzes the following:

$$H_2O + CO_2 \xrightleftharpoons[\text{anhydrase}]{\text{Carbonic}} H_2CO_3 \leftrightarrow H^+ + HCO_3^-$$

How does HCO_3^- enter the plasma?

Cl^- antiporter in RBC membrane (chloride shift)

Which two factors determine arterial or alveolar CO_2 tensions.

1. Rate of CO_2 production
2. Alveolar ventilation

What is the Haldane effect?

Binding of O_2 to hemoglobin reduces its affinity for CO_2

Where does the Haldane effect occur physiologically?

Lungs

What is methemoglobin?

Hb that contains ferric (Fe^{3+}) has a very high affinity for oxygen, resulting in decreased ability of Hb to unload oxygen.

How do obstructive diseases affect gas exchange?

Increases the time constant and result in a slower rate of alveolar filling and emptying

How do restrictive diseases affect gas exchange?

Reduce the time constant

PULMONARY CIRCULATION

What is the function of bronchial circulation?	Supplies the bronchotracheal tree with oxygen-rich arterial blood
Where does the bronchial circulation arise?	From the descending aorta or intercostal arteries (variable)
What percent of the left ventricular cardiac output does the bronchial circulation represent?	Roughly 2%
Where does the bronchial circulation drain?	Some to the azygous and hemiazygous systems, some directly to the pulmonary vein. Those going to the pulmonary vein comprise the physiologic shunt.
Compare pulmonary versus systemic circulation.	Pressures and resistance are much lower in the pulmonary circulation
How does pulmonary vascular resistance (PVR) compared with systemic resistance (SVR)?	PVR is about one-tenth of systemic resistance
What happens to resistance as pressure in the pulmonary artery increases?	Resistance decreases even lower because previously collapsed capillaries open up (recruitment) and individual capillary segments widen (distension)
What factors contribute to the large compliance of the pulmonary arterial tree?	Short pulmonary arterial branches All pulmonary arteries have larger diameters than their counterpart systemic arteries Vessels are very thin and distensible
At which point is the pressure in the pulmonary artery equal to the pressure in the right ventricle?	During the systolic phase of the cardiac cycle
What are the average pulmonary arterial pressures?	Systole: 25 mm Hg (compare with 120 mm Hg) Diastole: 8 mm Hg (compare with 80 mm Hg)

When supine, how is blood flow distributed, superiorly to inferiorly?

Equally (although the posterior aspects of the lung will have more perfusion)

When standing, how is blood flow distributed, superiorly to inferiorly?

There is increased flow to the bases (Zone 3) when compared to the apices (Zone 1)

What is responsible for this phenomenon?

Gravity

How is the pulmonary wedge pressure obtained?

Via a catheter introduced via the systemic venous circulation (e.g., femoral vein) that is *wedged* in a pulmonary arteriole

What does the pulmonary wedge pressure estimate?

1. Pulmonary venous pressure
2. Left atrial pressure (indirectly)
3. Left ventricular end-diastolic pressure (indirectly)

What happens when pressure in the pulmonary artery increases?

Resistance falls because of the recruitment phenomenon. Previously collapsed capillaries, distend and parallel capillary circuits are recruited.

What is the physiologic response of the lungs to hypoxia?

Vasoconstriction (opposite from the systemic response to hypoxia!)

Why does this occur?

To shunt blood away from non-ventilated regions of the lungs toward ventilated regions

What changes does chronic hypoxia cause in the pulmonary circulation?

Sustained pulmonary vasoconstriction

Increase in number of perivascular smooth muscle cells

Increased interstitial collagen

What are some consequences of long-standing pulmonary hypertension?

Cor pulmonale and right ventricular failure

How does inspiration affect venous return?

Increases it by increasing intrapleural pressure

VENTILATION AND PERFUSION

Define ventilation (*V*):	Transport of gas from the environment to the alveoli for gas exchange (normal about 4-6 L/min)
Define perfusion (*Q*):	Pulmonary blood flow to the alveolar capillaries
What is the normal *V/Q* ratio?	0.8 to 1.2
What is the most common cause of hypoxemia?	*V/Q* mismatch
What occurs to alveolar gas partial pressures with an increase in *V/Q*?	Decrease in P_{CO_2}, increase in P_{O_2}
What occurs to alveolar gas partial pressures with a decrease in *V/Q*?	Increase in P_{CO_2}, decrease in P_{O_2}
In other words, which area of the lung has greater dead space?	The apices; they are ventilated, but are poorly perfused.
What is the normal distribution of ventilation and perfusion in a standing person?	Ventilation: highest at base, lowest at apex Perfusion: highest at base, lowest at apex
Which has a higher *V/Q*: bases or apices?	Apices (ventilation > perfusion)
Which has a lower *V/Q*: bases or apices?	Bases (perfusion > ventilation)
Why is the *V/Q* ratio low at the base and high at the apex?	The change in blood flow from the apex to the base is *relatively greater* than the change in ventilation
What is a shunt?	Perfusion with no/low ventilation

In the following figure identify the area of highest perfusion and the area with the greatest dead space.

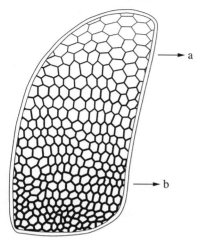

Figure 4.6 Ventilation and perfusion in the zones of the lung. (Reproduced, with permission, from Levitsky MG: *Pulmonary Physiology.* 7th ed. New York, NY: McGraw-Hill; 2007.)

a. Most dead space
b. Greatest perfusion

What is the Alveolar-arterial (A-a) gradient?	The discrepancy between alveolar and arterial oxygen partial pressures
What is the normal A-a gradient?	5 to 15 mm Hg
How is the A-a gradient calculated?	$PAO_2\ PaO_2 = P_1O_2 - \left(\dfrac{PaCO_2}{R}\right) - PaO_2$ PAO_2 = alveolar PO_2 PaO_2 = arterial PO_2 P_1O_2 = PO_2 of inspired gas $PaCO_2$ = arterial PCO_2 R = gas constant
What is responsible for the normal A-a gradient?	Regional V/Q mismatching Physiologic shunt Diffusion limitation (very small amount)
At what V/Q ratio does the most efficient gas exchange occur?	1:1, the oxygen in 1 liter of inspired air is best paired with 1 liter of blood

What causes low *V/Q*?	Inadequate ventilation (cessation of breathing, airway obstruction, etc)
What is the result of low *V/Q*?	An intrapulmonary shunt (perfusion without ventilation)

RESPIRATORY CONTROL

Where is respiration centrally controlled?	Reticular formation in the medulla (medullary respiration center)
Where do the nerve fibers that mediate inspiration converge?	On the phrenic motor neurons located in the ventral horns from C3 to C5 and the external intercostal motor neurons in the ventral horns throughout the thoracic cord
Where do fibers concerned with expiration converge?	Primarily on the internal intercostal motor neurons in the thoracic cord
What is the dorsal respiratory group (DRG)?	Inspiratory cells that may act as the primary rhythm generator for respiration
What stimulates DRG activity?	1. Low O_2 tensions 2. High CO_2 tensions 3. Low pH levels 4. Increased electrical traffic resulting from renal artery stenosis (RAS)
What nerves mediate input to the DRG?	Vagus: peripheral chemoreceptors and lung mechanoreceptors Glossopharyngeal: peripheral chemoreceptors
Where does the outflow from DRG project?	Contralateral phrenic and intercostals motor neurons, and the ventral respiratory group (VRG)
What makes up the VRG?	Upper motor neurons of the vagus and the nerves to the accessory muscles of respiration
What is the role of the VRG?	Activated to control expiration when it is an active process (e.g., exercise)

Where is the apneustic center?	Caudal area of the lower pons
What is the significance of the apneustic center?	Efferent outflow increases the duration of inspiration
Where is the pneumotaxic center?	Upper part of the pons
What is the function of the pneumotaxic center?	Unknown, it is thought to inhibit the apneustic center and shortens inspiration. It may play a role in switching between inspiration and expiration.
How does damage to the pneumotaxic center affect respiration?	Respiration becomes slower and V_T greater
Where are central chemoreceptors located?	Beneath the ventral surface of the medulla
What do central chemoreceptors respond to?	H^+ concentration in the cerebrospinal fluid (CSF) and the surrounding interstitial fluid
What is the major chemical drive of respiration?	CO_2 (H^+) effects on the central chemoreceptors
Where are the peripheral chemoreceptors located?	Carotid and aortic bodies
What do peripheral chemoreceptors respond to?	1. Lowered O_2 tensions 2. Increased CO_2 tensions 3. Increased H^+ concentrations in arterial blood
What stimuli affect the respiratory center?	Chemical control: 1. CO_2 (via CSF and brain interstitial fluid H^+ concentration) 2. O_2 (via carotid and aortic bodies) 3. H^+ (via carotid and aortic bodies) Nonchemical control: 1. Vagal afferents from receptors in the airways and lungs 2. Afferents from the pons, hypothalamus, and limbic system 3. Afferents from proprioceptors 4. Afferents from baroreceptors
Define apnea:	Cessation of respiration lasting > 20 seconds

What is obstructive sleep apnea (OSA)?	Recurrent interruptions of breathing during sleep due to temporary obstruction of the airway by lax, excessively bulky, or malformed pharyngeal tissues (soft palate, uvula, and sometimes tonsils), with resultant hypoxemia and chronic lethargy
How does OSA differ from central sleep apnea?	OSA: obstruction with respiratory effort (e.g., chest movement) Central sleep apnea: apnea without respiratory effort

RESPONSE TO STRESS

How does the respiratory system respond to exercise?	Increase minute ventilation (through initially increased tidal volume and then increased frequency) A-a gradient widens (excessive exercise) Respiratory (CO_2/O_2) exchange ratio exceeds 1, but < 1.25
How does the pulmonary blood flow change during exercise?	Increases, due to increased pulmonary artery pressures and a decrease in pulmonary vascular resistance (as well as more venous return to the heart due to deeper inspirations)
What occurs to the V/Q matching during exercise?	V/Q increases (ventilation increases more than perfusion increases)
How does the amount of O_2 in the body change with exercise?	Total O_2 content increases, but Pa_{O_2} remains steady
How does the P_{O_2} of blood flowing into the pulmonary capillaries change with exercise?	Falls to 25 mm Hg or less because of increased extraction
How does CO_2 excretion change with exercise?	Increases to as much as 40-fold because of increased amount of CO_2 produced
What happens to the mean values for arterial P_{O_2} and P_{CO_2} during exercise?	No change in oxygen, CO_2 constant during aerobic respiration (decreases slightly with anaerobic respiration and lactic acid production).

What happens to the level of lactate in the blood with exercise?	It increases
Where does lactate come from?	Muscles in which aerobic resynthesis of energy stores cannot keep pace with their utilization and an oxygen debt is incurred
What happens to arterial pH during exercise?	No change with moderate exercise, but it decreases with strenuous exercise due to lactic acidosis
What is hypoxia?	O_2 deficiency at the tissue level
What are the signs of hypoxia?	Cyanosis, tachycardia, and tachypnea
What are the symptoms of chronic hypoxia?	Dyspnea (the *feeling* of being shortness of breath)

CLINICAL VIGNETTES

A 4-year-old child accidentally inhales a French fry which moves down into the bronchial tree. The areas distal to the French fry are now deprived of ventilation. What does the body do to help ensure the best V/Q matching?

The arterioles that deliver deoxygenated blood to those alveoli which are now obstructed constrict shunting blood toward areas that are still well ventilated

A 46-year-old plumber presents to the doctor with slowly progressing difficulty breathing. He is diagnosed with restrictive lung disease secondary to exposure at work. How would his lung compliance be affected? Which part of breathing would he have difficulty with, inspiration or expiration? How would his FEV_1/FVC be affected?

His compliance would be decreased due to stiffness of his lungs. He would have trouble with inspiration, as the stiffness of his lungs would prevent him from expanding his lungs fully. His FEV_1/FVC would be unchanged, as his FEV_1 and FVC would be decreased in the same proportion.

A healthy, 25-year-old friend of yours asks you why exercise makes you feel short of breath. What is your answer?

You explain to him that during exercise, the limiting factor in oxygenation to tissues is not the amount of oxygen you are getting into your lungs, rather it is because of the amount of blood traversing the pulmonary vasculature per unit time (flow limitation). The body demands O_2 in excess of what is being delivered and central receptors perceive this as shortness of breath

A patient experiences shortness of breath of sudden onset after a long plane ride. After a spiral CT scan, she is diagnosed with a pulmonary embolism in a branch of a pulmonary artery. How are her pulmonary artery and vein pressures affected, respectively?

Her pulmonary artery pressure would increase (due to increased resistance), but her pulmonary vein pressure are unchanged, these are determined by left atrial pressures

Which obstructive lung disease causes a reduction in diffusing capacity of the lung for carbon monoxide (DLCO)?

Emphysema; as lung tissue is destroyed, less surface area exists to allow for diffusion

A 65-year-old male with a 75-pack-year smoking history presents to the pulmonologist for evaluation of his dyspnea and exercise intolerance. What values does the pulmonologist expect to see on his pulmonary function tests (PFTs)?

↓ forced expiratory volume (FEV_1)

↓ FEV_1/forced vital capacity (FVC)

↑ total lung capacity (TLC)

A 60-year-old heavy smoker presents to the doctor with long-standing shortness of breath, especially upon exertion. She is diagnosed with emphysema. How are her FEV_1 and RV impacted by this disease process?

Her FEV_1 would be markedly reduced, and her RV would be increased as she is having trouble expiring.

A patient who is experiencing daytime somnolence presents to his physician. His physician describes sleep apnea. What test would be ordered to definitively diagnose the patient?

A sleep study would be performed

A healthy, 30-year-old man ascends Mt Everest. As he ascends, he begins to feel dyspneic. What is the cause of his shortness of breath? What will he do acutely to compensate for his altitude change? What chronic changes will occur to compensate for his altitude change?

His shortness of breath is due to a decreased ambient PO_2 because of decreased atmospheric pressures. Acutely, there is an increase in respiratory rate (leading to a respiratory alkalosis), increase in tidal volume and a total increase in alveolar ventilation. Chronically (i.e., acclimatization) there is renal compensation for the alkalosis as well as increased erythropoiesis to increase the oxygen-carrying capacity of the blood.

A 45-year-old female with severe scoliosis and no history of tobacco use complains of dyspnea. What category of lung disease does she have?

Restrictive lung disease, thoracic cavity changes impair her ability to expand her lungs.

A 40-minute-old male neonate of an 18-year-old Caucasian female at 27 weeks gestation is noted to have central cyanosis. His respirations are shallow and rapid at 65/min. Other vital signs are stable. On examination, there is nasal flaring, audible grunting, and duskiness with intercostal and subcostal retractions. Fine rales are heard over both lung bases. Nasal O_2 does not improve his cyanosis. A chest x-ray (CXR) reveals fine reticular granularity, predominantly in lower lobes. Arterial blood gas (ABG) reveals hypoxemia with metabolic acidosis. What is the underlying cause of his condition?

Decreased production and secretion of surfactant resulting in atelectasis and shunting (perfused but non-ventilated alveoli). This ventilatory defect leads to the bodies inability to excrete its acid load

How do the PFTs in a patient with restrictive scoliosis differ from those with parenchymal disease and associated restrictive disease?

DLCO is normal in a patient with scoliosis, whereas it is reduced in a patient with parenchymal disease

A 34-year-old male presents to his PCP with cough, rhinitis, and wheezing. The patient had missed his appointment for similar symptoms 3 weeks ago, stating he felt better after spending his 3-day weekend resting. The patient has been working in a textile dye factory for the past 9 months. He presents today with reportedly worsening cough and difficulty breathing over the last week. He almost cancelled today's appointment because his symptoms seemed better having rested over the weekend. What is the probable diagnosis based on this patient's history?

Occupational asthma; repeated exposure to certain substances (called sensitizers) can lead to immune sensitization.

In this case, the dyes at work have become the offending agent, but things like latex, molds seen in agriculture and detergents have also been known to cause these types of scenarios.

What test can be used to aid in the diagnosis of the above patient?

Measure peak expiratory flow (PEF) and correlate changes with workplace exposure

What class of antihypertensive drugs should patients with asthma avoid?

Nonselective beta-blockers (e.g., metoprolol, atenolol)

A 67-year-old woman (height: 65 in, weight: 110 lb) with a known history of systemic lupus erythematosus (SLE) presents with progressively nonproductive cough and increasing dyspnea on exertion. She denies weight loss, fever, and hemoptysis. On pulmonary examination, respiratory rate (RR) 26 and faint bibasilar rales are appreciated. PFTs: FVC 3.1 (59%), FEV_1 2.2 (56%), maximum voluntary ventilation (MVV) 90 L/min, DLCO 14 mL/min/mm Hg (44%). A CXR reveals increased linear markings at the bases bilaterally. Based on the patient's history and PFTs, what property of the lungs is most likely affected?

Compliance is decreased from her restrictive lung disease

In the patient above, an ABG at room air was obtained as follows: pH 7.44, Pa_{O_2} 60 mm Hg, and Pa_{CO_2} 35 mm Hg. What is the alveolar to arterial oxygen gradient?

$$A\text{-a gradient} = F_iO_2(P_{atm} - P_{water\ vapor}) - (Pa_{O_2} + Pa_{CO_2}/R)$$
$$A\text{-a} = 21\%(760 - 47) - (60 + 35/0.8)$$
$$A\text{-a} = 45.9, \text{ a large gradient}$$

A 51-year-old man with known interstitial lung disease with resting ABG: pH 7.45, Pa_{O_2} 60 mm Hg, and Pa_{CO_2} 30 mm Hg. After walking on a treadmill for 5 minutes, another ABG was drawn with a Pa_{O_2} 52 mm Hg and Pa_{CO_2} 30 mm Hg. What is the most likely mechanism for the worsening hypoxemia observed postexercise?

Abnormalities in diffusion. In a patient with interstitial lung disease where the lung parenchyma is affected, diffusion of oxygen often becomes an issue. That is, O_2 stops being a "perfusion limited" gas, and becomes a "diffusion limited" gas

A 66-year-old woman with chronic obstructive pulmonary disease (COPD) presents to the ED with progressively worsening dyspnea and a chronic cough. On physical examination, the patient was noted to have bibasilar rhonchi, diffuse wheezing bilaterally, and decreased breath sounds. A CXR reveals large hilar shadows suspicious for large pulmonary arteries and right atrial enlargement, which was also seen on ECG. What does this patient likely have?

Pulmonary hypertension secondary to chronic COPD.

In these patients the loss of alveolar septae also destroys small pulmonary vasculature thereby eliminating vessels from parallel circuits. This loss increases total pulmonary resistance.

A young man is in a motor vehicle accident in which he suffers trauma leading to the paralysis of his diaphragm. What changes will occur in his blood gases from his injury?

It causes global hypoventilation:

pH decreased

Pa_{O_2} decreased

Pa_{CO_2} increased

A-a gradient is unchanged

What is the most common cause of hypoxemia encountered in the clinical setting?

Ventilation-perfusion mismatch

A 22-year-old tall healthy male presents with sudden new-onset sharp chest pain and dyspnea. He denies any recent fevers or coughs. He also denies trauma to the chest. He is markedly tachypneic. A CXR reveals a moderate-sized pneumothorax at the left apex and no other abnormalities. What happened to the patient's lung and chest wall in this condition?

The lung collapsed inward away from the chest wall; this is common in tall Caucasian males and is caused by pleural "blebs" which rupture releasing air into the pleural space

How does carbon monoxide poisoning affect arterial O_2 concentration?

Decreases it, but, use caution when evaluating patients at the bedside, the Hb-CO complex is detected by pulse oximeters as being saturated and can mislead clinicians.

A 67-year-old male with a 100-pack-year history of smoking presents to the ED with progressively worsening dyspnea. On examination, the patient appears barrel-chested. He is visibly gasping for air with pursing lips and using his accessory muscles. Lung examination reveals wheezing and coarse stridorous breath sounds. Pulse oximetry shows O_2 saturation of 86%. The patient is given a breathing treatment as well as oxygen therapy. Why must oxygen therapy be administered with caution in this patient who is in severe respiratory distress?

This patient most likely has severe COPD from his extensive smoking history. It is likely that he is also hypercapnic, in which case, the patient may be dependent on his hypoxic drive (via the carotid and aortic chemoreceptors) to stimulate respiration as opposed to the usual CO_2 level. If the hypoxic drive is withdrawn by administering O_2, the patient may become apneic, causing the arterial PO_2 to drop and increase PCO_2. Breathing may not restart because the increase in PCO_2 will further depress his respiratory center.

How does anemia affect PO_2?

Decreases mixed-venous PO_2

An elderly patient, hospitalized for knee replacement surgery, was found on postop day 5 with a 1-day fever, productive cough, and upper airway congestion. A CXR reveals localized infiltrates in the right middle lobe suggestive of pneumonia. What would the resting ABG look like if one were to be obtained?

The patient is expected to have shunting due to probable pneumonia:

1. pH increased
2. PaO_2 decreased
3. $PaCO_2$ decreased
4. A-a gradient is widened

Hypoxemia due to shunt does not respond to increased FiO_2.

CHAPTER 5

Renal and Acid–Base Physiology

BODY FLUIDS

Explain the 60-40-20 rule.	Total body water (TBW), in liters, is 60% of body weight in kilograms, intracellular fluid (ICF) is 40% of body weight, and extracellular fluid (ECF) is 20% of body weight
What is the distribution of ECF in the human body?	ECF is one-third of TBW. Plasma is one-fourth of ECF or one-twelfth of TBW. Interstitial fluid is three-fourths of ECF or one-fourth of TBW.
What are the major cations of the ICF and ECF?	ICF: K^+ and Mg^{2+} ECF: Na^+
What are the major anions of the ICF and ECF?	ICF: protein and organophosphates ECF: Cl^- and HCO_3^-
What substance is used to measure the following major fluid compartments?	
TBW	Tritiated H_2O or D_2O
ECF	Sulfate, inulin, or mannitol
Plasma	Radioiodinated serum albumin (RISA), Evans blue
Interstitial fluid (IF)	*Indirectly*: IF = ECF − plasma
ICF	*Indirectly*: ICF = TBW − ECF

What is the method for using the above listed substances to calculate these volumes?

The dilution method. A known amount of substance is administered to your patient and then given time to equilibrate in the volume of interest. Now if we collect a sample and again determine its concentration, we can calculate that volume.

$$C_1 \times V_1 = C_2 \times V_2$$

C_1 = concentration of injected substance

V_1 = volume of injected substance

C_2 = concentration of measured sample

V_2 = value to be calculated

RENAL BLOOD FLOW AND FILTRATION

What percentage of the cardiac output goes to the kidneys?

20%; the highest blood flow of any organ when calculated per gram tissue.

Describe the blood flow through the glomerulus:

Blood enters via the renal arteries and is shuttled through large arteries to the afferent arterioles. It then flows through the glomerular tuft and out into an efferent arteriole (*not* a venule).

Once blood passes through the efferent arteriole where does it go?

This efferent flow provides blood to the peritubular capillary beds, with some going to the vasa recta. Very little of the total renal blood flow (RBF) moves through the vasa recta.

What is autoregulation of RBF?

Process by which renal vasculature changes resistance to keep the glomerular blood flow and filtration pressures consistent.

Describe the hypothesized mechanisms by which autoregulation is achieved:

Myogenic mechanism: stretch receptors in renal arterioles detect rising pressures and cause the contraction of the afferent arterioles, to increase resistance, and maintain constant blood flow.

Tubuloglomerular feedback: the macula densa senses [Na^+] changes and uses that as a measure of filtrate flow rate. It directs the afferent arterioles to change its resistance thereby changing flow.

What inflammatory cytokine is important in dilating the afferent arteriole?

Prostaglandins. These are used in the signaling pathway for vessel dilation. This is one of the reasons why the use of nonsteroidal anti-inflammatory drugs is dangerous in people with kidney disease who rely on higher filtration pressures to maintain GFR.

What hormone is important in constricting the efferent arteriole?

Angiotensin II. The use of ACE or ARB class antihypertensive drugs can be dangerous in patients with poor renal function, as it can reduce glomerular filtration pressures.

What are the components of the glomerular filtration barrier?

Fenestrated capillary endothelium

Fused basement membrane lined with heparan sulfate

Epithelial layer consisting of podocyte foot processes

Bowman's space

Podocyte foot processes

Glomerular basement membrane

Fenestrated capillary epithelium

Capillary lumen

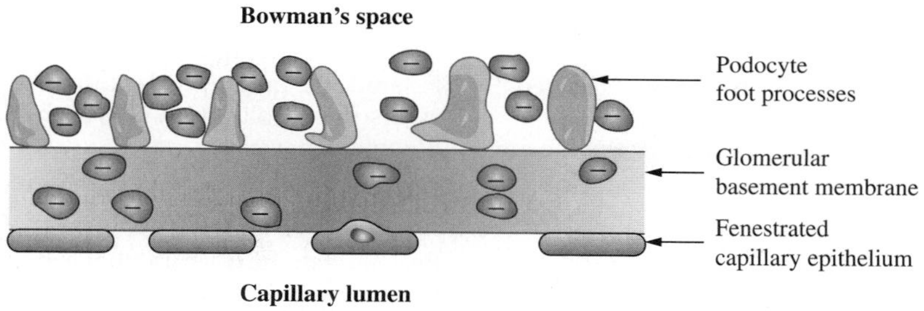

Figure 5.1   Anatomy of the renal filtration system.

What is the purpose of the fenestrated endothelium?

This is a very coarse filter and really only impedes RBC from moving out of the vessel

What does the basement membrane do?

It offers a "size barrier" to plasma proteins restricting all but the smallest proteins to the vascular space

What aspect of the filtration barrier prevents the smallest proteins from entering Bowman space?

Anionic glycoproteins (heparan sulfate) that line the basement membrane repel the negatively charged proteins ("charge barrier")

What is "clearance"?

In physiology, it is the volume of plasma that is cleared (cleaned, if you will) of a substance per unit time.

What is the equation used to measure clearance (C) of the kidney?

$$C = \frac{U \times V}{P}$$

C = clearance
U = urine concentration of substance x
V = urine flow rate
P = plasma concentration of substance x

In words, what is the glomerular filtration rate (GFR)?

GFR is the volume of plasma per unit time that moves from the vascular space to Bowman space.

What can be used clinically to approximate GFR?

Creatinine (Cr) clearance

What makes creatinine clearance so well-suited to use in the clinical setting?

It is endogenously produced as a product of muscle turnover at a consistent rate for a given muscle mass, and it is filtered readily at the glomerulus and only minimally secreted or reabsorbed in the nephron

What is meant by the terms "filtered," "secreted," and "reabsorbed"?
(we will return to this ad nauseum below)

Filtered: the quantity of solute that enters the tubular fluid (TF) at the Bowman space

Secreted: the quantity that is put into the TF as it moves through the nephron

Reabsorbed: the quantity that is removed from the TF and put back into the plasma

What substance is used to measure renal plasma flow (RPF)? Why?

Para-aminohippuric acid (PAH), it is filtered *and* secreted by renal tubules (so it gives us a measure of *all* blood moving through the kidney, not just the filtered fraction). Note that this is a research tool, primarily

How is RPF calculated?

RPF is measured as the clearance of PAH

$$RPF = C_{PAH} = \frac{[U]_{PAH} \times V}{[P]_{PAH}}$$

C_{PAH} = clearance of PAH
$[U]_{PAH}$ = urine concentration of PAH
V = urine flow rate
$[P]_{PAH}$ = plasma concentration of PAH

How do you measure renal blood flow (RBF)?

$$RBF = \frac{RPF}{(1 - \text{hematocrit})}$$

What is the filtration fraction (FF)?

The fraction of renal plasma flow that moves into Bowman space

How is FF calculated?

$$FF = \frac{GFR}{RPF}$$

What is the normal value for FF?

Under physiologic conditions, one-fifth of RPF is filtered at the glomerulus, or about twenty percent.

What happens to the protein concentration in the peritubular capillaries with increasing FF?

Increases; as filtrate is removed in the glomerulus the remaining blood products become more concentrated

What substance is used to *definitively* measure the glomerular filtration rate (GFR)? Why?

Inulin: it is filtered but not reabsorbed or secreted by the renal tubules, also primarily a research tool

What equation is used to directly measure GFR?

Using the clearance equation with inulin

$$GFR = C_{inulin} = \frac{[U]_{inulin} \times V}{[P]_{inulin}}$$

C_{inulin} = clearance of inulin

$[U]_{inulin}$ = urine concentration of inulin

V = urine flow rate

$[P]_{inulin}$ = plasma concentration of inulin

How does falling GFR effect blood urea nitrogen (BUN) and plasma Cr?

Causes them to increase, since both are filtered by the glomerulus

Does GFR remain constant with aging?

No, it decreases with age

What happens to plasma Cr with age?

It remains relatively constant despite the decrease in GFR with age due to the decrease in muscle mass seen with aging. Less muscle means less turnover.

What is the Starling equation for GFR?

$$GFR = K_f \left[(P_{GC} - P_{BS}) - (\pi_{GC} - \pi_{BS}) \right]$$

Describe each of the following terms from the Starling equation:

K_f

Filtration coefficient across the glomerular barrier.

P_{GC}

Hydrostatic pressure in the glomerular capillary. This is essentially the blood pressure of the glomerular capillaries and is determined by the resistance of the afferent and efferent arteriole.

P_{BS}

Hydrostatic pressure in Bowman space, under normal physiologic conditions, this value should be very low.

π_{GC}

Oncotic pressure in the glomerular capillary. It increases along the length of the glomerular capillary as filtrate is removed from the capillary.

π_{BS}

Oncotic pressure in Bowman space, since protein is kept within the capillary, this value should be zero.

What can cause an increase in P_{GC}? What is the effect on GFR?

Dilation of the afferent arteriole or constriction of the efferent arteriole. This elevated hydrostatic pressure will increase GFR.

What can cause an increase in P_{BS}? What is the effect on GFR?

Any obstruction of the tubules or of the lower urinary tract. This increased pressure decreases GFR.

In a patient with cirrhosis, who has lost some hepatic synthetic capacity (fewer serum proteins), how is the π_{GC} changed?

This will reduce the oncotic pressure, and increase the GFR

If the urine concentration of inulin is 0.25 mg/mL, the urine flow rate is 25 mL/min and the plasma concentration of the drug is 0.12 mg/mL, what is the renal clearance?

Using the equation for clearance

$U = 0.25$ mg/mL

$V = 25$ mL/min

$P = 0.12$ mg/mL

$$C = \frac{0.25 \text{ mg/mL} \times 25 \text{ mL/min}}{0.12 \text{ mg/mL}}$$

$C = 52$ mL/min

RENAL SECRETION, REABSORPTION, AND EXCRETION

Identify the portions of the nephron numbered in the diagram below.

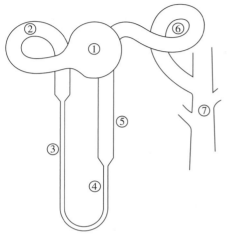

1. Bowman space
2. Proximal tubule
3. Descending limb of the loop of Henle
4. Thin ascending limb of the loop of Henle
5. Thick ascending limb of the loop of Henle
6. Distal convoluted tubule
7. Collecting duct

Figure 5.2   Nephron structure.

How is the elimination rate of a given substance calculated?

$$E_y = (FL_y + S_y) - R_y$$

E_y = Elimination rate of substance y

FL_y = Filtration rate of substance y

S_y = Secretion rate of substance y

R_y = Reabsorption rate of substance y

How is the rate at which a molecule is filtered across the glomerular capillary calculated?

$$FL_y = GFR \times P_y$$

FL_y = Filtered load of substance y

P_y = Substance plasma concentration

How is the rate of a molecule's excretion in urine calculated?

$$E_y = U_y \times \dot{V}$$

E_y = Excreting rate of substance y

V = Urine flow rate

U_y = Concentration of substance in urine

How do you determine if a substance is ultimately secreted or absorbed?	Take the difference between rate excreted and rate filtered (excreted-filtered): If > 0 → secretion If < 0 → absorption If = 0 → neither secreted nor absorbed
Will secreted substances have higher or lower clearance rates than the filtration rate?	Higher
Will reabsorbed substances have higher or lower clearance rates than the filtration rate?	Lower
If we plot filtration and excretion rates across many plasma concentrations, what do we generate?	Renal titration curves. These can be plotted for any renally handled substance.
As an example, let us consider glucose:	
Is glucose normally secreted or reabsorbed?	Reabsorbed
How?	There are very efficient Na^+-glucose cotransporters found in the proximal tubules which mediate glucose uptake
At what concentration of glucose does the Na^+-glucose carriers in the proximal tubules start to become saturated? What happens to any glucose above this level?	Approximately 250 mg/dL; once this level is exceeded some glucose begins to spill into the urine as the cotransporters become saturated. At 350 mg/dL glucose uptake is saturated and all increases in filtered glucose will be excreted
What is it called when the kidney *begins* to excrete a substance that should be conserved (250 mg/dL for glucose)?	Renal threshold, above this point, glucose transport in some of the nephrons is saturated, so glucose begins to appear in urine.
What is the term for the glucose concentration where the maximum rate of solute transport is achieved?	Transport maximum (T_m). Note that different sources will give you different values for threshold and T_m.

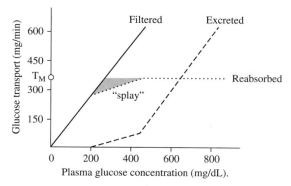

Figure 5.3   Glucose titration curve.

What is splay?	The region on a titration curve between the renal threshold and T_m. In this region some nephrons have maximized their transport capacity for glucose, others, because of larger population of transporters, have not.
What is the splay for glucose?	Between 250 to 350 mg/dL

As another example, let us look at the renal handling of PAH:

What happens to the filtered load of PAH as the plasma load of PAH increases?	Increases in direct proportion to the plasma load
Is PAH secreted or reabsorbed?	Secreted
Where does this occur?	Proximal tubules
What is the mechanism by which PAH is secreted?	Specialized carriers in the proximal tubules mediate transcellular transfer of PAH into the tubular fluid (TF).
What happens to secretion of PAH when T_m is reached?	It plateau's and any further increase in plasma PAH will not change the secretion rate
How is excretion calculated for PAH (and other secreted substances)?	We modify the elimination formula to calculate PAH excretion. Since PAH is filtered and secreted, but not reabsorbed, the formula simplifies to:

$$E_{PAH} = (FL_{PAH} + S_{PAH})$$

When using PAH to measure RBF, what important limitation must be appreciated?

RPF can only be measured at plasma concentrations $< T_m$

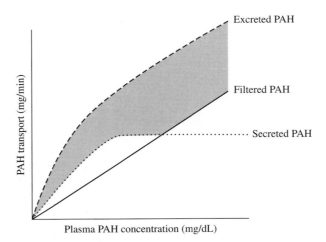

Figure 5.4   Titration curve for PAH.

PAH, then, has a very high elimination rate that approaches 100%. What are some examples of substances with very low elimination rates?

Na$^+$

Glucose

Amino acids

HCO$_3^-$

Cl$^-$

What does the ratio of $[x]_{TF}$ to $[x]_P$ represent (i.e. the TF/P ratio)?

It compares the concentration of a substance in TF with that of plasma

What is the utility of this value?

It allows us to interpret renal handling of a given substance; that is, does the body want to get rid of it, hold on to it, etc.

What does each of the following ratios represent?

TF/P = 1

Either there is no reabsorption of the substance or reabsorption of the substance is equal to that of water

TF/P < 1

Reabsorption of a substance is greater than water, thus concentration of substance x in TF is less than plasma

TF/P > 1

Reabsorption of a substance is less than water, thus concentration of substance x in TF is greater than plasma

What substance can be used as a marker for water reabsorption along the nephron and why?

Inulin.

Because inulin is freely filtered, but it is neither secreted nor reabsorbed, so its concentration in TF changes only as a consequence of water reabsorption

Na⁺ and K⁺ Handling

In renal water management, what is the primary electrolyte that we pay attention to clinically?

Sodium (Na^+); "water always follows salt"

Give the percentage of Na⁺ reabsorption along the following parts of the nephron:

Proximal convoluted tubule (PCT)	67%
Thin descending limb	0%
Thin ascending limb	0%
Thick ascending limb	25%
Distal convoluted tubule (DCT)	5%
Collecting ducts (CDs)	3%

What percentage of all of the filtered Na⁺ is excreted in a normal nephron?

1% to 2%, depending on an individual's total salt intake

In the early proximal tubule, what major substances are preferentially reabsorbed with Na⁺ by cotransport?

Glucose

Amino acids

Phosphate

Lactate

Which one of these coupled solutes is most important for Na⁺ recovery?

No one solute; they all play an important role in the sodium handling of the proximal tubule.

How is HCO_3^- reabsorbed in the proximal tubule?

Via carbonic anhydrase, which converts it to CO_2 that can move transcellularly. This is the solute that gets the most attention in the proximal tubule, likely because it's the one that we can most potently influence pharmacologically.

At physiologic values, what percentage of glucose and amino acids are reabsorbed in the proximal tubule?

100%

Is Na⁺ reabsorbed at a constant or variable rate in the proximal tubule?

Essentially constant; 67% of all filtered Na⁺ is reabsorbed

What is the name of the mechanism by which this is accomplished?

Glomerulotubular balance

What forces influence glomerulotubular balance?

The same Starling forces that balance fluid filtration at the glomerulus also influence the peritubular capillary blood vessels. It works to balance glomerular filtration.

What is the effect of the following on reabsorption?

(Think: Starling forces)

Increased GFR
Increased FF

Increased: in both cases, the removal of more plasma volume at the glomerulus results in hemoconcentration and a resultant increase in protein concentration

ECF volume contraction

Increased: by increase in peritubular protein concentration and decrease in peritubular pressure

ECF volume expansion

Decreased: by decrease in peritubular protein concentration and increase in peritubular pressure

Describe the mechanism by which Na⁺-H⁺ exchange occurs in the proximal tubule:

Na⁺ is reabsorbed by coupled exchange with H⁺. This process is directly linked to HCO_3^- reabsorption (see below).

What brush border enzyme is responsible for the Na⁺/HCO_3^- reabsorption mechanism?

Carbonic anhydrase

Generally speaking, how is Na⁺ reabsorbed in the late proximal tubule?

Na⁺ is reabsorbed with Cl⁻, although the various segments use different transporters to accomplish this.

What happens in the descending limb and the thin ascending limb of the loop of Henle?

There is no net reabsorption of water here; the movement of water and electrolytes helps to generate an osmotic gradient in the medulla of the kidney (more later)

What transporter is responsible for reabsorption of Na⁺ in the thick ascending limb of the loop of Henle?

Na⁺-K⁺-2Cl⁻ cotransporter in the luminal membrane

What diuretics are responsible for inhibition of this transporter?

Loop diuretics: furosemide, ethacrynic acid, and bumetanide

Is the thick ascending limb of the loop of Henle permeable to water?

No, therefore, NaCl is reabsorbed without water thereby diluting the tubular fluid.

What happens to the osmolarity of the TF and [Na⁺] in the thick ascending limb compared to plasma?

Decreases, which is why the segment is called the *diluting segment*

What change can be seen in transluminal electrical potential in this segment?

The luminal fluid gains a slight net positive charge; the Na-K-2Cl cotransport removes two negative and two positive charges making transport electroneutral.

However, a luminal K⁺ channel (the *romK* channel) allows for backleak of positive charge across the luminal membrane leading to a net positive tubular fluid (more on this in *other e-lytes*)

Why is this luminal positive charge important?

It is important in establishing a driving force for paracellular cationic efflux from the tubular fluid (Ca⁺⁺, Mg⁺⁺, etc.)

What transporter is responsible for Na⁺ reabsorption in the early distal tubule?

Na⁺-Cl⁻ cotransporter

What diuretics work on the transporter in this segment?

Thiazide diuretics

Is the early distal tubule permeable to water?

No

What happens to the osmolarity of the solution in the tubular lumen in this section?

It becomes further diluted

Name the cell types responsible for electrolyte transport in the late distal tubule and CDs.

Principal cells and α-intercalated cells

In principal cells, what major electrolytes are secreted and which are reabsorbed?

Secreted: K^+
Reabsorbed: Na^+ and H_2O

What is the other important hormone that influences principal cells?

ADH (vasopressin)

How does ADH work?

It directs the insertion of water channels (aquaporins) into principal cell luminal membranes

What effect does aldosterone have on electrolyte reabsorption or secretion?

Increases Na^+ reabsorption and K^+ secretion

What percentage of overall Na^+ reabsorption is affected by aldosterone?

2%, but this is the important 2% that fine tunes sodium balance

What diuretics work on principal cells?

K^+-sparing diuretics (spironolactone, triamterene, amiloride), which block sodium channels and sodium channel insertion preventing sodium reabsorption and, indirectly, decreasing K^+ secretion

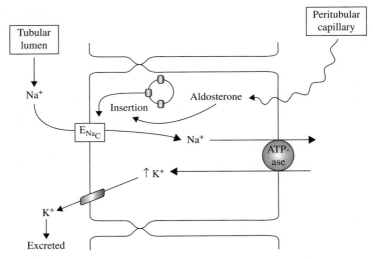

Figure 5.5   Principal cell. (Note the sequestered $E_{Na}C$ that are inserted into the luminal membrane with aldosterone stimulation.)

What is the major function of the α-intercalated cells?

Contributes to acid-base management

What electrolytes are secreted and reabsorbed in α-intercalated cells?

Secreted: H^+ (by H^+-ATPase)

Reabsorbed: K^+ (by H^+-K^+-ATPase)

What influence does aldosterone have on α-intercalated cells?

Increases H^+ secretion by directly stimulating H^+-ATPase activity

Give the equation to calculate fractional excretion of sodium (Na^+) (FENa).

$$FENa = \frac{Urine[Na^+] \times Plasma[Cr]}{Plasma[Cr] \times urine[Na^+]}$$

What conditions are associated with the following values of FENa?

<1%

Hemodynamic causes of renal failure (most commonly volume depletion). This indicates that the body is avidly retaining sodium, and therefore water

>1%

Clinical conditions which disrupt the usual mechanisms of sodium reabsorption; commonly, acute tubular necrosis (ATN) but also bladder stone or bilateral ureteral obstruction

What are the values for FENa and urine [Na^+] that are suggestive of prerenal azotemia?

FENa < 1%

Urinary Na^+ < 20 mEq/L

What are the values for FENa and urine [Na^+] that are suggestive of ATN or postrenal azotemia?

FENa > 3%

Urinary Na^+ > 40 mEq/L

Clinically, diuretic use can perturb the interpretation of FENa, so what other urinary solute can be used?

Urea, but note that the values used to interpret it differ significantly.

Generally speaking, how does the kidney handle K^+?

It is finely regulated. In general, the proximal nephron reabsorbs K^+ while the distal nephron uses aldosterone to fine tune the amount of excreted K^+.

Where is most of the body's K^+ located?

ICF

Name some factors that lead to K^+ entering cells.

Insulin

β-Adrenergic agonists

Alkalosis

Name some factors that lead to cellular efflux of K⁺.

Insulin deficiency (e.g., diabetes)

β-Adrenergic antagonists

Acidosis

Cell lysis

Exercise

Na^+-K^+ pump inhibitors

Give the percentages for K⁺ reabsorption along the various parts of the nephron.

PCT	67%
Thin descending limb	0%
Thin ascending limb	20%
Thick ascending limb	Variable
DCT	Variable
CDs	Variable

What percentage of filtered K⁺ is excreted in a normal nephron?

1% to 110% (extremely variable based on dietary intake)

How is K⁺ reabsorbed in the thick ascending limb?

By the Na^+-K^+-$2Cl^-$ cotransporter, but recall that most of it leaks back into tubular fluid to generate the transcellular gradient

How is K⁺ reabsorbed in the distal tubule and CDs?

By the H^+-K^+-ATPase in the luminal membranes of α-intercalated cells

What is the mechanism of distal K⁺ secretion in the basolateral and luminal membranes?

Basolateral: Na^+-K^+-ATPase pump (active)

Luminal: K^+ channels (passive)

How do each of the following conditions affect K⁺?

Mentally review the reason and mechanism.

High K⁺ diet	Increase secretion
Low K⁺ diet	Decrease secretion
Hyperaldosteronism	Increase secretion
Hypoaldosteronism	Decrease secretion
Acidosis	Decrease secretion
Alkalosis	Increase secretion
Thiazide and loop diuretics	Increase secretion
Increased luminal anions	Increase secretion
Spironolactone, triamterene, amiloride	Decrease secretion (K⁺-sparing diuretics)

How does aldosterone affect K⁺ secretion in the kidney?

↑ aldosterone secretion
↓
Aldosterone leads to Na⁺ channel (ENaC) insertion in principal cells
↓
↑ Na⁺ entry across luminal membrane into the cells
↓
↑ activity of Na⁺-K⁺ pump on the basolateral membrane
↓
↑ Na⁺ secretion out of the cells and ↑ K⁺ cell entry across basolateral membrane
↓
↑ intracellular [K⁺]
↓
↑ K⁺ secretion across luminal membrane

Describe the pathway by which acidosis affects K⁺ secretion:

↑ blood H⁺
↓
↑ H⁺ entry across basolateral membrane
↓
↑ K⁺ egress across basolateral membrane
↓
↓ intracellular K⁺
↓
↓ K⁺ secretion across luminal membrane (Hyperkalemia)

Describe the pathway by which alkalosis affects K⁺ secretion:

↓ blood H⁺
↓
↓ H⁺ entry across basolateral membrane
↓
↓ K⁺ secretion across basolateral membrane
↓
↑ intracellular K⁺
↓
↑ K⁺ secretion across luminal membrane (reverse of acidosis)

Describe the mechanism by which thiazide and loop diuretics affect K⁺ secretion:

↑ flow rate through distal tubule
↓
Dilution of luminal [K⁺]
↓
↑ driving force for K⁺ secretion

What diuretic is a direct antagonist to aldosterone?	Spironolactone; it competes with the hormone receptor found *inside* the principal cell
How do triamterene and amiloride work?	They antagonize the inserted ENaC channel.

UREA, MG^{++}, CA^{++}, AND HPO$_4^{2-}$ HANDLING

Urea is produced as a product of what biologic process?	Nitrogen metabolism, largely due to processing of proteins
How is nitrogen measured clinically?	Plasma [BUN]
Where is the majority of urea reabsorbed?	50% is passively reabsorbed in the proximal tubule
What parts of the kidney are impermeable to urea?	Distal tubule Cortical CDs Outer medullary CDs
How is urea handled in the loop of Henle?	It is reabsorbed into the interstitium where it generates the osmotic gradient for water reabsorption in the collecting tubules
Calcium regulation involves primarily what three organs?	Intestines → absorption Kidney → excretion Bone → long-term storage
What percentage of total plasma Ca^{2+} is filtered across the glomerular capillaries? Why?	~60%; Calcium circulates in three forms, ionized, or unbound calcium, bound to proteins, some large, some small, and complexed with small anionic molecules. Ionized calcium is readily filtered, as are some small anionic compounds, but most protein bound calcium (40%) is not.
Where is the majority of Ca^{2+} reabsorbed?	Proximal tubule and thick ascending limb
Is Ca^{2+} reabsorbed in the distal tubule?	Yes, this is where parathyroid hormone (PTH) primarily works. PTH stimulates the activity of the apical Ca^{2+} channel, but this accounts for only a fraction of total renal Ca^{2+} handling.

As a rule, calcium follows another cation with respect to segmental handling, what anion is that, and what is the segmental exception to the rule?

Calcium generally follows sodium in the way it is handled on a segmental basis, the CD, though, does not allow for calcium reabsorption

What percentage of calcium reabsorption takes place in the distal tubule?

8%

What diuretics can be used in hypercalcemia?

Loop diuretics; by blocking the Na-2Cl$^-$-K cotransporter, a less positive luminal charge exists, which decreases the driving force for Ca^{++} reabsorption. This increases urinary excretion of calcium

What diuretics can be used in hypercalciuria (like with calcium based kidney stones)?

Thiazide diuretics; by blocking the distal tubules Na$^+$-Cl$^-$ cotransporter, the distal nephron increases Ca^{++} (an alternate cation) reabsorption

What diuretics decrease Ca^{2+} excretion?

Thiazide diuretics, see above question for mechanism

How much of the body's total phosphate load is found free in the ECF?

Less than 1%

Where in the body is the majority of it found?

In bone and intracellular fluid

Where in the kidney is the majority of phosphate reabsorbed?

Typically, 80% is reabsorbed in the proximal tubule (with ~20% excreted)

How is phosphate reabsorbed in the kidney?

By Na$^+$-phosphate cotransporter

What renal parameter most influences renal phosphate handling?

GFR. Since ~80% of phosphate is reabsorbed in the proximal tubule, a falling GFR results in reduced phosphate reabsorption.

What effect does increased [phosphate]$_{plasma}$ have on PTH release?

PTH release is increased

How does parathyroid hormone affect phosphate regulation in the kidney?

Inhibits its reabsorption in the proximal tubule by inhibiting the Na$^+$-phosphate cotransporter

What parts of the kidney play a role in Mg^{2+} reabsorption?

Proximal tubule

Thick ascending limb

Distal tubule

What electrolyte competes with Mg^{2+} for reabsorption in the thick ascending limb?

Ca^{2+}, again, Ca^{2+} and Mg^{2+} move paracellularly driven by changes in luminal charge. The pathway can only accommodate so many ions.

How does hypercalcemia affect Mg^{2+} reabsorption?

It decreases Mg^{2+} reabsorption, and thereby increases Mg^{2+} excretion

DILUTION AND CONCENTRATION OF URINE

In water deprivation, what part of the brain is activated?

Osmoreceptors in the anterior hypothalamus

Do peripheral baroreceptors influence ADH secretion?

Yes, but to a much smaller degree

What is the primary stimulus for ADH release?

Increased plasma osmolarity

What part of the brain secretes ADH?

Posterior pituitary

Name some states associated with high levels of circulating ADH.

Hemorrhage

Water deprivation

Syndrome of inappropriate antidiuretic hormone (SIADH)

What is the corticopapillary osmotic gradient?

Osmolar gradient that exists from the renal cortex to the papilla

What are the primary electrolytes responsible for creating the corticopapillary osmotic gradient?

NaCl and urea

How is the gradient established?

Countercurrent multiplication and urea recycling

Describe the countercurrent multiplication in a kidney with high circulating ADH.

NaCl is reabsorbed in the thick ascending limb while there is countercurrent flow in the descending and ascending limbs of the loop of Henle, amplifying the osmotic concentration of the interstitium

What hormone augments countercurrent multiplication in the kidney?	ADH: stimulates NaCl reabsorption in the thick ascending limb thereby increasing the size of the gradient
What is urea recycling?	Process by which urea goes from the inner medullary CDs into the medullary interstitial fluid
What hormone augments urea recycling?	ADH
How is the urea gradient maintained in the kidneys?	Countercurrent exchange

In the figure below, describe what is happening in the five labeled steps?

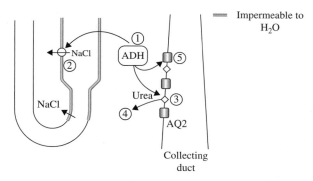

Figure 5.6   ADH and osmotic gradient.

Step 1	High plasma osmolarity leads to increased $[ADH]_{plasma}$
Step 2	Medullary osmotic gradient is increased as NaCl reabsorption in the thick ascending limb (TAL) is stimulated (increased countercurrent multiplication)
Step 3	Urea cycling activity also increases between the medulla and the inner medullary collecting ducts
Step 4	Net effect: high medullary osmotic pressure
Step 5	ADH leads to insertion of aquaporin 2 channels, water moves down its gradient and is taken back into circulation

What are the vasa recta?

Capillary network surrounding the loop of Henle in the renal medulla.

How do vasa recta affect countercurrent exchange?

They serve as osmotic exchangers. The blood in them tries to equilibrate osmotically with the interstitial fluid in the medulla and papilla.

What about the vasa recta blood flow is unique?

In order to prevent equilibration these vessels deliver a lower volume of blood to a slower flowing circuit. This helps to prevent osmotic washout.

What would happen if blood flow were too great?

The blood would carry away all of the osmotically active solutes that the above system is set up to put there.

What parts of the nephron are impermeable to water?

Thin and thick ascending limb of the loop of Henle and early distal tubule

What parts of the kidney increase reabsorption of water in the presence of ADH?

Late distal tubule and CDs

What protein, when ADH stimulation is present, is inserted in the principal cells that allows for water transport out of the tubular fluid?

Aquaporin 2

What happens to ADH with decreased plasma osmolarity?

Secretion is inhibited

Name some conditions that are associated with very low levels of circulating ADH.

Excess water intake and central diabetes insipidus; interestingly ethanol also suppresses ADH secretion

What is the osmolarity without ADH and with high levels of ADH in the following regions of the nephron?

	High ADH	No ADH
Proximal tubule	300 mOsm/L	300 mOsm/L
Thick ascending limb	100 mOsm/L	120 mOsm/L
Early distal tubule	90 mOsm/L	110 mOsm/L
Late distal tubule	300 mOsm/L	100 mOsm/L
CDs	1200 mOsm/L	50 mOsm/L

What formula is used to estimate the ability to concentrate or dilute urine?	Free-water clearance (C_{H_2O}) $$C_{H_2O} = V - C_{osm}$$ V = urine flow rate (mL/min) C_{osm} = osmolar clearance
What is "free water clearance"?	It is the rate at which the kidney absorbs or excretes water in excess of solute
What does a positive value for (C_{H_2O}) mean?	Excess water excretion: urine is hypotonic to plasma (absence of ADH)
What does a negative value for (C_{H_2O}) mean?	Decreased water excretion: urine is hypertonic to plasma (high ADH)

ACID-BASE

What is the normal pH of plasma?	7.35 to 7.45
What is the origin of our acid burden?	Metabolism
How does the body transport H^+ ions through the body?	CO_2, a volatile acid
How does CO_2 transport allow for H^+ ion transport?	$$H_2O + CO_2 \xrightleftharpoons{\text{Carbonic anhydrase}} H_2CO_3 \leftrightarrow H^+ + HCO_3^-$$
What enzyme allows this reaction to proceed?	Carbonic anhydrase
Name some *nonvolatile* acids generated by the body.	Phosphoric acid Ketoacids Lactic acid
What three mechanisms are used by the body to help insulate against pH disturbance?	1. Ventilatory changes 2. Buffers 3. Renal H^+ excretion/HCO_3^- retention
What are buffers?	Compounds that prevent large changes in pH with the addition or loss of H^+ ions
In general, what types of compounds make the best buffers?	Weak acids and bases
Why do they make the best buffers?	They are stable compounds with pK values close to normal pH which are well suited to accepting/releasing H^+ ions

With respect to pK_a, when are buffers most effective?

When they are within 1 pH unit of their pK

What is the major extracellular buffer? What is its pK?

Bicarbonate (HCO_3^-), pK_a = 6.1

What is a minor extracellular buffer? What is its pK?

Phosphate, pK = 6.8

What is the most important buffer in urine?

Phosphate

What does titratable acidity mean relative to the human urine?

Amount of NaOH required to neutralize a 24-hour urine specimen back to pH of 7.4

What are the titratable acids used by the body?

$H_2PO_4^-$, H_2SO_4

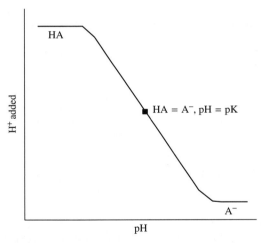

Figure 5.7   Weak acid titration curve.

In the figure above, where on the curve is the buffer most effective?

On the steep portion of the curve. Large concentration changes are equal to only small pH changes.

What is important about the part of the graph where concentrations of HA and A⁻ are equal?

pH = pK

How does ventilatory change influence a patient's acid-base status?

It allows the body a minute-to-minute tool to eliminate or conserve volatile acid: CO_2

How does hyperventilation influence the body's acid-base status?

This decreases total acid load. Increasing minute ventilation increases CO_2 loss.

Does acidosis or alkalosis have a greater influence over ventilation?

Acidosis; we are better able to increase minute ventilation to expel more CO_2 than we are able to decrease it. Decreasing it can compromise our ability to oxygenate.

If someone has an acute respiratory acidosis, how much do we expect the pH to fall?

For each rise in pCO_2 of 10, the pH will fall by .08

What if that respiratory acidosis goes on for a while (becomes chronic)?

The pH will reflect a .04 fall for every 10 mmHg increase in pCO_2

In what two ways does the kidney help to regulate acid-base balance?

1. Regulation of plasma $[HCO_3^-]$
2. Excretion of metabolic acids

Where is the majority of filtered HCO_3^- reabsorbed?

Proximal tubule

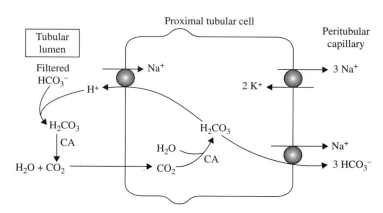

Figure 5.8 HCO_3^- reabsorption.

In the process of HCO_3^- reabsorption are H^+ ions secreted or reabsorbed?

Neither, they are recycled and reused for bicarbonate recovery

In fact, in conditions of acidosis, what cannot happen to urine until bicarbonate recovery is complete?

The urine cannot be acidified. Until bicarbonate is removed the tubular fluid cannot hold onto excess hydrogen ions because they are preferentially used for bicarbonate recycling.

Describe how Pco_2 affects HCO_3^- reabsorption?

Increases in Pco_2: increases rates of HCO_3^- reabsorption because the supply of intracellular H^+ increases

Decreases in Pco_2: decreases rates of HCO_3^- reabsorption because the supply of intracellular H^+ decreases

Describe how ECF volume affects HCO_3^- reabsorption?

$\uparrow$ ECF volume: $\downarrow$ HCO_3^- reabsorption
$\downarrow$ ECF volume: $\uparrow$ HCO_3^- reabsorption (also due to secretion of angiotensin II)

Describe how angiotensin II affects HCO_3^- reabsorption?

Stimulates the Na^+-H^+ countertransporter, which leads to increase in H^+ secretion into the urine resulting in increased HCO_3^- generation.

How is H^+ secreted in urine?

Attached to titratable acids and as NH_4^+

How much, as a percent, of the kidneys H^+ ion excretion is in the form of ammonia?

~75%

What do renal cells use to produce NH_3?

Glutamate

Describe the process of renal ammoniagenesis:

Mitochondria in the proximal tubule deaminate glutamate, which is then transported into the tubular lumen.

What other by-product of that reaction influences acid-base balance?

It produces two new HCO_3^- ions.

What two factors influence H^+ excretion as NH_4^+?

1. NH_3 produced by the renal tubular cells
2. Urine pH

How does NH_3 get transported in the urinary lumen?

Down its concentration gradient by simple diffusion; NH_3 is highly membrane *permeable*

What does the term *diffusion trapping* mean?

H^+ is secreted separately and combines with NH_3 to form NH_4^+, which *traps* the H^+ in the tubular fluid promoting excretion. NH_4^+ is membrane *impermeable*.

What happens to excretion of NH_4^+ at lower pHs?

Increased excretion because there is a greater ratio of NH_4^+ compared to NH_3

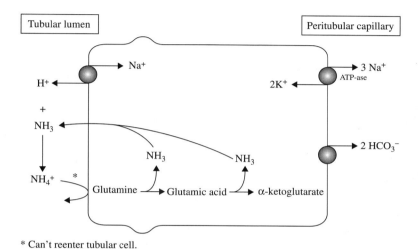

* Can't reenter tubular cell.

Figure 5.9   Renal ammoniagenesis. The NH_4^+ molecule is "stuck" in the tubular lumen due to it's charge.

What happens to NH_3 synthesis in acidosis?

Increases

What is the primary disturbance in each of the following conditions?

    Metabolic acidosis

Gain of nonvolatile acids, or loss of bicarbonate

    Metabolic alkalosis

Usually from loss of endogenous hydrogen ions (vomiting, for example)

    Respiratory acidosis

Hypoventilation

    Respiratory alkalosis

Hyperventilation

Describe the respiratory response in each of the following conditions:

Metabolic acidosis

Hyperventilation, while it doesn't get rid of the nonvolatile acids that are accumulating, it does lower total acid load by eliminating CO_2

Metabolic alkalosis

Hypoventilation

Describe the renal compensation in each of the following conditions:

Acute respiratory acidosis

Minimal

Chronic respiratory acidosis

$\uparrow$ H^+ excretion (by eliminating NH_4^+) and $\uparrow$ HCO_3^- reabsorption

Respiratory alkalosis

$\downarrow$ HCO_3^- reabsorption

What is Kussmaul breathing?

Hyperventilation secondary to acidemia

Describe Kussmaul breathing.

Patients are taking very fast, but very deep breaths, thus increasing their minute ventilation. This allows patients to better eliminate CO_2.

What adaptation occurs in states of chronic metabolic acidosis?

Increase in both HCO_3^- and NH_3 synthesis, for reclamation and secretion, respectively.

What is Winter's equation?

Expected $pCO_2 = 1.5 \times [HCO_3^-] + 8 \pm 2$

How do we use Winter's equation clinically?

It allows us to evaluate compensation in metabolic acidosis.

We enter the value for HCO_3^-, and the resulting number should be ± 2 of the patient's pCO_2 if there is appropriate compensation.

What is the equation for serum anion gap (AG)?

$AG = [Na^+] - ([Cl^-] + [HCO_3^-])$

What does the value for AG represent?

Unmeasured anions in serum

Give some examples of unmeasured anions.

Phosphate, Citrate, Lactate, Sulfate, Formate, Methanol, Formaldehyde

What is the normal range for the AG?

8 to 12 mEq/L

What is the mnemonic for causes of anion gap metabolic acidosis?

MUDPILES
Methanol
Uremia (from chronic renal failure)
Diabetic ketoacidosis
Paraldehyde/Phenformin
Iron/Isoniazid (INH)
Lactic acidosis
Ethanol/Ethylene glycol
Salicylates

List some conditions that result in non-anion gap metabolic acidosis.

1. Diarrhea
2. RTA types 1, 2, and 4

What is the mnemonic for *non-anion gap* metabolic acidosis?

HARDUP
Hyperalimentosis
Acetazolamide
Renal tubular acidosis
Diarrhea
Ureteroenteric fistula
Pancreaticoduodenal fistula

List some conditions that result in metabolic alkalosis.

Vomiting
Hyperaldosteronism
Loop and thiazide diuretics

Volume contraction is a common cause of metabolic alkalosis. Why?

The nephron, in its eagerness to increase plasma volume, tries to reclaim anything that passes through it, this includes bicarbonate.

How can diuretics cause metabolic alkalosis?

By volume contraction, through the above mechanism

How does vomiting lead to metabolic alkalosis?

H^+ is lost in vomitus combined with volume contraction

List some conditions that may result in respiratory acidosis.

Guillain-Barré syndrome
Polio
Amyotrophic lateral sclerosis (ALS)
Multiple sclerosis (MS)
Airway obstruction
Acute respiratory distress syndrome (ARDS)
Chronic obstructive pulmonary disease (COPD)

List some substances associated
with respiratory acidosis.

Opiates

Sedatives

Anesthetics

List some conditions that result
in respiratory alkalosis.

Pneumonia

Pulmonary embolus

High altitude

Psychogenic

Salicylate intoxication

Within the physiologic pH range,
is deoxyhemoglobin or oxyhemoglobin
a better buffer?

Deoxyhemoglobin

CLINICAL VIGNETTES

A 58-year-old woman comes to your laboratory for a study which demands that
you know the volume of plasma in her body.

What substance should you use?

Radioiodinated serum albumin (RISA) or Evans blue

If we inject 1000 mg of RISA, which has a concentration of 1 mg/mL, and allow
it to equilibrate, and then find it has a concentration of 0.303 mg/mL, what is her
total plasma volume?

$$C_1 \times V_1 = C_2 \times V_2$$

X = 1000mg/0.303 mg/mL (where X is plasma volume)

X = 3300 mL

Plasma volume = 3.3 L

A 4-year-old boy is brought into your office. His mother tells you that he has been
swelling for the past day or so, but this morning his face became very puffy and
she is very concerned. Laboratory examination reveals 4+ (profound) protein in the
urine. What aspect of kidney filtration has failed?

The protein barrier is made up of both a size and a charge filter. The size filter
protects from loss of large proteins, but small proteins, notably albumin, can sneak
through. The charge filter defends against those smaller proteins. This boy is
losing albumin excessively because of charge filter failure.

The following values were found while studying an isolated glomerulus: afferent arteriole pressure = 30 mm Hg, oncotic pressure of glomerular capillary = 25 mm Hg, Bowman space pressure = 12 mm Hg. From these values, determine whether filtration will be favored or not.

Net pressure is determined from the Starling equation by excluding the filtration constant, and recognizing that π_{BS} is zero.

The equation can be written as: net pressure = $(P_{GC} - P_{BS}) (\pi_{GC} - 0)$

Plugging the numbers in $(30 - 12) - (25) = -7$ mm Hg

A negative value indicates that filtration is not favored. Normally a positive number represents a net pressure that favors filtration, because the forces promoting filtration outweigh those forces that oppose filtration.

A 54-year-old man comes to your office for routine follow-up. He has been on spironolactone for a year but has recently noticed that he has had some enlargement in his breast tissue (gynecomastia). You decide that you would like to use a similar drug that doesn't have that particular side effect. What diuretics work directly on the principal cell *channels*?

Triamterene and amiloride; these drugs are Na^+ channel blockers that selectively target the ENaC channel on the principal cells luminal membrane.

Using the following diagram, describe how the body's water composition changes in the give situations:

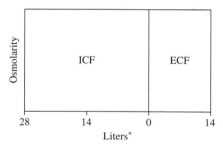

*Values based on 70 kg patient

Figure 5.10   Fluid compartments.

(These questions show up all over the boards, get familiar with them now.)

A young woman comes into the office after just returning from a trip to Mexico for her spring break. On her last day there she ate some food from a roadside vendor and developed isotonic diarrhea. What immediate changes will you see in the fluid distribution?

Diarrhea: extracellular fluid (ECF) decreases with no change in osmolarity. There is no change in the volume of the intracellular fluid (ICF).

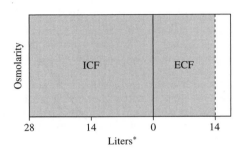

Figure 5.11   Diarrhea.

Some eager medical students want to prepare for their clinical rotations and decide to practice giving injections of isotonic saline to a willing volunteer. What immediately happens to the fluid compartments as they do this?

Infusion of isotonic saline: the osmolarity of the fluid is the same compared to that of the body fluids, so it mostly stays in the ECF. Thus the volume of the ECF increases with no change in the ICF.

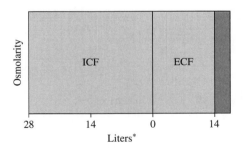

Figure 5.12   Isotonic saline.

You go to your friend's house for the biggest sporting event of the year. He has all sorts of salty party food and you dig right in. Unfortunately the water to his apartment has been turned off, he's got nothing to drink in his fridge, and no one is willing to leave the game to get some drinks. What is happening to your fluid compartments?

Excessive NaCl intake: this increases the osmolarity of the ECF, thus drawing the fluid out of the ICF into the ECF. The result is a decrease in volume of the ICF and increase in volume of the ECF, while increasing the osmolarity of both ICF and ECF.

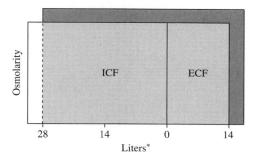

Figure 5.13   Excess NaCl.

A young lady has been recently diagnosed with adrenal insufficiency. Please draw the diagram and describe the situation.

Adrenal insufficiency: results in a loss of NaCl, thus ECF osmolarity decreases and the volume of the ECF also decreases. As a result, water diffuses into the ICF until the osmolarity of ICF and ECF are equal, raising the volume of the ICF and decreasing of the ECF.

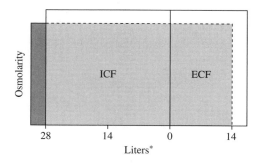

Figure 5.14   Adrenal insufficiency.

A young woman who has recently been diagnosed with oat cell cancer of the lung comes into the office because she is feeling drowsy. Physical examination shows a hypertensive patient with dry mucous membranes, poor skin turgor, peripheral edema, and crackles in the base of the lungs. Routine laboratory results show sodium of 123. A diagnosis of syndrome of inappropriate antidiuretic hormone (SIADH) is made. What is the fluid versus osmolarity body composition of a patient with SIADH? Explain why.

SIADH: this causes retention of free water by the kidneys, which results a net decrease of osmolarity of the both ICF and ECF. Slightly more fluid goes into the ICF compartment because it is a larger space.

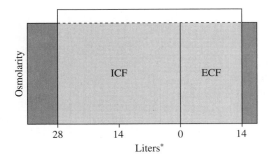

Figure 5.15 SIADH.

A second-year medical student is studying for his USMLE Step 1 when the air conditioner breaks in his apartment. It is a hot spring day and the student begins to sweat. It is Sunday and the library is closed, so the diligent student stays in his hot apartment and studies all day despite the heat. He forgoes drinking fluids to maximize his study time. Describe the change of his body fluid dynamics and why it occurs.

Sweating: sweat has more water than salt, so there is a net hyperosmotic volume contraction. ECF volume decreases, water shifts out of ICF leading to increased ICF osmolarity until it is equal to ECF osmolarity. As a result of all of this, there is still a net ICF and ECF volume loss with increased osmolarity of ICF and ECF.

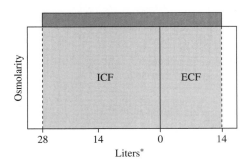

Figure 5.16 Sweating.

A man has been on trip to Mexico. After he returns, he goes to his doctor with severe diarrhea. An ABG shows the following values: pH = 7.2, P_{CO_2} = 25, [HCO_3^-] = 8 mEq/L. Further lab values find Na^+ to be 135 and Cl^- to be 118. What is the anion gap? What acid-base disorder does this patient suffer from?

$$\text{Anion gap} = [Na^+] - ([Cl^-] + [HCO_3^-])$$
$$= 135 - (115 + 8) = 12$$

This is a normal anion gap. With a low pH, we know that it is either metabolic or respiratory acidosis. Since the P_{CO_2} is normal and the HCO_3^- is low, it is a metabolic acidosis likely secondary to his diarrhea.

A woman, complaining of frequent urination and occasional headaches, visits her doctor for further workup. Her plasma osmolarity is found to be 270 mOsm/L and urine osmolarity 1200 mOsm/L. What is the diagnosis for this patient?

SIADH. The plasma osmolarity is lower than normal, yet the urine osmolarity is still high. The body should be maximally *diluting* the urine, not concentrating. These findings are indicative of SIADH.

A volunteer is injected with para-aminohippuric acid (PAH) to measure renal plasma flow (RPF). Plasma concentration of PAH is 2 mg/mL, urine concentration of PAH is 500 mg/mL, and urine flow rate is 1 mL/min. What is the RPF?

Using the equation:
$$RPF = C_{PAH} = ([U]_{PAH} \times V)/[P]_{PAH}$$
$$RPF = (500 \text{ mg/mL} \times 1 \text{ mL/min })/2 \text{ mg/mL} = 250 \text{ mL/min}$$

In the above patient, the hematocrit is found to be 40%. What is the renal blood flow? What is an approximation of the cardiac output in this patient?

$$\text{Renal blood flow (RBF)} = RPF/(1 - \text{hematocrit})$$
$$RBF = 250/(1 - 0.4) = 250/0.6 = 416.67 \text{ mL/min}$$

RBF is ~20% of cardiac output. So, RBF = CO × 0.2 or CO = RBF/0.2 = 2083.4 mL/min

A middle-aged man comes to the ER complaining of 10/10 stabbing left-sided flank pain that started early in the morning. He does not report any fever or chills. On ultrasound, he is found to have a ureteral stone. What is the effect of this ureteral stone on glomerular filtration rate (GFR), RPF, and filtration fraction (FF)?

GFR will decrease because of the increased pressure in Bowman space (obstruction means higher pressures upstream). There will be no change in RPF because there is no change in the blood flow to or from the kidneys. The filtration fraction will decrease because GFR has decreased and RPF has remained unchanged.

A recently discovered drug (drug X) has been found to have a side effect of causing constriction of afferent renal arterioles. What will be the effect on the FF?

It will be unchanged! Even though there will be a decrease in RPF, there will also be a decrease in GFR from drop in P_{GC}.

A young woman comes to the doctor after being treated for a bad urinary tract infection. Her GFR is found to be 100 mL/min. Her plasma glucose level is found to be 150 mg/dL and urine glucose concentration level is found to be 1000 mg/dL with flow at 3 mL/min. Determine whether there is net absorption or secretion of glucose.

$$\text{Rate filtered} = \text{GFR} \times \text{Plasma [glucose]}$$
$$= 100 \text{ mL/min} \times 150 \text{ mg/dL}$$
$$= 150 \text{ mg/min}$$
$$\text{Rate secreted} = \text{V} \times \text{urine [glucose]}$$
$$= 3 \text{ mL/min} \times 1000 \text{ mg/dL}$$
$$= 30 \text{ mg/min}$$
$$\text{Difference} = 150 - 30 = +120 \text{ mg/min}$$

Therefore, glucose is reabsorbed.

What commonly used cardiac drug can cause hyperkalemia (high K^+)? How?

Digitalis—blocks the Na^+-K^+ pump meaning that less K^+ is made intracellular

What happens to the urinary secretion of Ca^{2+} in a person on loop diuretics (e.g., furosemide)?

Increases (loop diuretics inhibit Na^+ reabsorption, which is coupled to Ca^{2+} reabsorption)

When someone drinks excess water, what happens to the osmoreceptors in the anterior hypothalamus? What does this lead to?

Inhibited. This causes the pituitary to release less ADH and, therefore, encourages the kidney to increase the free water clearance.

What is a condition in which antidiuretic hormone (ADH) is ineffective?

Nephrogenic diabetes insipidus; in this condition ADH is released but the collecting ducts are not responsive to its effects

What medication may cause ADH to become ineffective?

Lithium

A 50-year-old woman presents to her doctor with tinnitus. During examination, she was found to have rapid breathing, and an ABG showed a P_{CO_2} of 24. Her laboratory results were found to be:

$Na^+ = 140$

$K^+ = 5$

$Cl^- = 105$

$HCO_3^- = 15$

$BUN = 43$

$Cr = 1.7$

1. Calculate the anion gap.
2. What *should* the compensatory pCO_2 be?
3. What are the acid-base disturbances?
4. What drug(s) can cause these types of disturbances?

Calculate serum anion gap:

$$Na^+ - (Cl^- + HCO_3^-) = \text{anion gap}$$
$$140 - (105 + 15) = 20$$

From this, we know that she has a metabolic acidosis, with an anion gap.

I like to use Winter formula to calculate the expected pCO_2:

$$Expectedp\ CO_2 = 1.5*HCO_3^- + 8 \pm 2$$

Using this equation you can determine that appropriate compensation will yield a pCO_2 of 29 to 33.

The lower P_{CO_2} than calculated indicates that she also has a respiratory alkalosis.

So, the drug most likely to cause both a respiratory alkalosis and metabolic acidosis is salicylate.

CHAPTER 6

Gastrointestinal Physiology

GENERAL FEATURES

In general, the gastrointestinal (GI) tract includes what structures?

The entire gut tube from mouth to the anus, as well as the accessory organs of digestion (liver, gallbladder, and pancreas)

What is the primary function of the GI (alimentary) tract?

Nutrient absorption

Gut motility refers to what?

The movement of food (in various stages of digestion) through the GI tract

What is the innermost surface of the gut tube?

The mucosa (composed of the first four items in the next question)

Please identify the labeled components of cellular anatomy in the following cross-section of the GI tract.

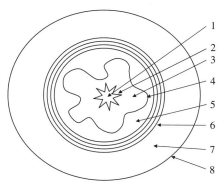

1. Lumen
2. Epithelial cells
3. Lamina propria
4. Muscularis mucosa
5. Submucosa
6. Circular muscle
7. Longitudinal muscle
8. Serosa

Figure 6.1 Structural features of the GI tract.

What is the main muscle type in the GI canal?

Visceral smooth muscle (VSM)

Where in the GI tract do we have skeletal muscle?

In the oropharynx and esophagus (absent by the distal third of the esophagus) where we have voluntary control over swallowing and chewing, and the external anal sphincter which we gain control of during infancy

What is unique about the muscle in the GI tract?

The smooth muscle cells are interconnected by gap junctions and function together as a single unit, much like cardiac muscle. Thus, an action potential generated in one muscle cell can easily spread to adjacent cells, allowing the cells to peristalse

Describe the roles of the following anatomical regions of the GI tract:

Oropharynx

Chewing breaks food into smaller pieces which provides more surface area for digestion, also houses some glands which begin secreting hydrolyzing enzymes

Esophagus

Propels food from oropharynx to stomach

Stomach

Grinds and mixes food with stomach acids to provide a suitable slurry to enter the small intestine

Small intestine

The workhorse of nutrient absorption; entry into small intestine is coordinated with the secretion of the various exocrine enzymes from the liver and the pancreas (more to come)

Large intestine

Water and electrolyte reabsorption along with storage of fecal waste

How long does transit through the following GI segments take?

Esophagus

Seconds

Stomach

2 to 5 hours, conventionally we talk about the stomach being 50% empty after 3 hours.

Small intestine

Also 2 to 5 hours

Large intestine

Approximately 30 to 50 hours

What is the collective term for the immune defense of the gut?	Gut-associated lymphoid tissues (GALT); this term encompasses a number of different lymphatic tissues throughout the gut tube
List some of the major component lymphatic tissues in the GI tract.	Tonsils, Peyer patches, lymphoid aggregate in the appendix

GASTROINTESTINAL CONTROL—NERVOUS

Name the two main nervous systems of the gut.	1. Enteric or intrinsic system 2. Autonomic or extrinsic system
What are the components of the extrinsic system? (Not including the control of the oropharynx)	Parasympathetic nervous system (PNS) and sympathetic nervous system (SNS)
Name the main function of the PNS in the GI tract.	Excitation
Which nerves carry PNS fibers and what structures/organs do they innervate?	Vagus: esophagus, stomach, pancreas, small intestine, and first portion of the large intestine Pelvic splanchnic nerves: second portion of large intestine, rectum, and anus
Name the main function of the SNS with respect to the GI tract.	Inhibitory
Which GI nerves carry SNS fibers?	Spinal nerves
Is the action of SNS exclusively inhibitory?	No
Where are the exceptions?	Lower esophageal sphincter, pyloric, and internal anal sphincter
Why does sympathectomy not affect alimentary motility?	Reuptake of norepinephrine (NE) by sympathetic nerve endings is so rapid that only a great rise in NE concentration during a sympathetic discharge can have a significant effect on normal GI motility
Overexcitation of the extrinsic nervous system can produce what common syndrome?	Irritable bowel syndrome (IBS)
What afferent information is carried by the extrinsic system?	All conscious sensations from the gut: fullness, pain, nausea, etc.

What are the two anatomical components of the intrinsic system?	Myenteric or Auerbach plexus Submucosal or Meissner plexus
What are the functions of the intrinsic system?	Acts as mediator of information between the extrinsic nervous system and the alimentary tract Commands most functions of the GI tube especially motility and secretion Can execute neural function of the gut without extrinsic innervations
Where is the myenteric plexus located?	It lies between the longitudinal and circular muscle layers
What is the main function of the myenteric plexus?	Controls and coordinates motility
Where is the submucosal plexus located?	It lies in the submucosa (hence the name), between the muscularis mucosa and circular muscle layer
What is the main function of the submucosal plexus?	Controls secretion and absorption as well as local blood flow

GASTROINTESTINAL CONTROL—HORMONAL

What is the main stimuli for hormone release?	Food lying adjacent to GI mucosa
What is the main function of GI hormones?	Regulate the digestive process by influencing secretion, motility, and blood flow
What are hormones? (see Chapter 7 for more details)	Chemical signals that fall into many categories, which help relay signals across varying distances
Define neurocrine.	Process in which one nerve fiber releases messenger that acts across a short distance upon a target cell (nerve fiber, muscle cell, or gland cell)
Define paracrine.	Released messenger acts upon adjacent cells
Define endocrine.	Stimulus acting upon a receptor causes the cell to release a messenger into the bloodstream that then acts on a distant target cell

Define neuroendocrine.

Action potential causes release of messenger that enters the bloodstream and acts upon a distant target cell

Name the main gastric hormones.

Gastrin

Cholecystokinin (CCK)

Secretin

Gastric inhibitory peptide (GIP)

Name the cells that secrete gastrin.

G cells in the antral mucosa of stomach

Of the above types of hormonal systems, which is used by gastrin to exert its effect?

Endocrine (and to a lesser degree neuroendocrine)

What are the three forms of gastrin?

1. Big gastrin (34 amino acids)
2. Little gastrin (17 amino acids)
3. Mini gastrin (14 amino acids)

Which form of gastrin is most abundant and potent?

Little gastrin

Which form has the longest half-life?

Big gastrin (42 minutes)

Which amino acids confer physiological activity?

Last four amino acids at the carboxy terminal (i.e., little gastrin: AA 14 to 17)

What are the major stimuli for gastrin's secretion?

1. Amino acids; notably L-amino acids like phenylalanine, tryptophan, cysteine, tyrosine
2. Vagal stimulation
3. Stomach distention

What are the functions of gastrin?

1. Primary: *Increases hydrochloric acid (HCl) secretion (via parietal cells)*
2. Stimulates growth of gastric mucosa
3. Increases gastric motility
4. Increases LES contraction (preventing reflux)
5. Decreases ileocecal sphincter contraction (dubbed the gastrocolic reflex; this allows defecation)
6. Increases pepsinogen secretion

What are some other stimuli for gastrin's secretion?

Epinephrine

Calcium

Acetylcholine (ACh)

What are the inhibitors of gastrin secretion.

pH < 2 (feedback inhibition)

Somatostatin

Secretin

Calcitonin

GIP

Glucagon

Vasoactive inhibitory peptide (VIP)

Which other GI hormone is chemically "related" to gastrin?

CCK, which shares five amino acids on the carboxy terminal, the extra amino acid of CCK offers receptor specificity, but cross activation is possible

While the two enzymes share five amino acids, how do they differ in their shared function?

Potency

What cells secrete CCK?

I cells of the duodenum and jejunum

Which hormonal system is used by CCK to exert its effects?

Endocrine

What are the major stimuli for CCK's secretion?

Protein and fat digestion products in the small intestine

What product of fat digestion does not stimulate CCK secretion?

Triglycerides

Why don't triglycerides stimulate the release of CCK?

They cannot cross the intestinal membranes

Which form is most abundant and potent?

CCK 8 (octapeptide)

On which amino acid sequence is the physiological activity located?

On the octapeptide on the carboxy terminal

What are the functions of CCK?

Increase gallbladder and pancreatic contraction

Decrease contraction of the sphincter of Oddi, allowing pancreatic secretion

Slow gastric emptying

Increase pepsinogen secretion

Decrease LES contraction

Stimulate growth of the exocrine pancreas

Work synergistically with secretin to increase bicarbonate secretion in the small intestine

What syndrome occurs when non-β-cell tumors of the pancreas secrete gastrin (e.g., gastrinoma)?

Zollinger-Ellison syndrome

Name the cells that secrete secretin.

S cells of the duodenum

What is the *primary* stimulus for secretin secretion?

H^+ in the duodenum

What is another stimuli for secretin release?

Protein and fat digestion products in the small intestine

What system of cellular communication is used by secretin to exert its actions?

Endocrine and paracrine

What are the functions of secretin?

1. Stimulates bicarbonate secretion from pancreatic and biliary duct cells
2. Decreases HCl secretion
3. Enhances activity of CCK on pancreatic secretion and gallbladder contraction
4. Decreases gastric and intestinal motility
5. Increases pepsinogen

Which hormones are part of the secretin-glucagon family?

Secretin

Glucagon

Vasoactive intestinal peptide (VIP), sometimes called vasoactive *inhibitory* peptide

Gastric inhibitory peptide (GIP)

What cells secrete GIP?

K cells of the jejunum and duodenum

What are the major stimuli for GIP's release?

Products of carbohydrate and fat breakdown in the small intestine

What system is primarily used by GIP to exert its actions?

Endocrine

What are the functions of GIP?

Stimulates insulin release and inhibits H^+ secretion

What are the GI paracrine hormones?

Somatostatin, serotonin, and histamine

Name the cells that secrete somatostatin.

Multiple cells in the GI tract

What is the stimulus for somatostatin release?

Presence of H^+ in the lumen

What inhibits the secretion of somatostatin?	Vagal stimulation
What is the function of somatostatin?	Think: "stasis" 1. Inhibits release of all GI hormones 2. Inhibits gastric H^+ secretion 3. Inhibits gallbladder and pancreatic contraction
Name the cells that secrete histamine.	Enterochromaffin-like (ECL) cells within the gastric mucosa
What is the function of histamine in the GI tract?	Increases gastric H^+ secretion (both directly and by potentiation of the effects of gastrin and vagal stimulation)
Why does that relationship make sense? (think about mast cell activation → increased acid secretion)	Histamine functions, in general as an immune cytokine, in the gut it has a similar function- acidification of the gastric lumen makes the environment far more hostile to arriving pathogens
What cells secrete serotonin?	Enterochromaffin (EC) cells in the gut wall
What is their primary stimulus for secretion?	Distension of the gut lumen
What does serotonin do in the gut?	It is primarily excitatory and leads to increased gut motility
What are the GI neurocrine hormones?	VIP Gastrin-releasing peptide (GRP) (bombesin) Enkephalins
What other GI hormone is VIP homologous to?	Secretin
Name the cells that normally secrete VIP.	Neuronal cells in the mucosa and smooth muscle of the GI tract
What tumor type can also secrete VIP?	Pancreatic islet cell tumors
What are the functions of VIP?	Relaxes GI smooth muscle (including LES) Stimulates pancreas to secrete HCO_3^- Inhibits gastric H^+ secretion

Name the cells that secrete GRP.	Vagal nerves that innervate G cells
What is the function of GRP?	Stimulates gastrin release
What are the types of enkephalins?	Met-enkephalin and Leu-enkephalin
Name the cells that secrete enkephalins.	Neurons in the mucosa and smooth muscle of the GI tract
What are the functions of enkephalins?	1. Contract GI smooth muscle (especially lower esophageal, pyloric, and ileocecal sphincters) 2. Inhibit secretion of fluid and electrolytes by the intestines
What hormone is secreted into the bloodstream to increase appetite?	Ghrelin
What is ghrelin's stimulus for secretion?	Hypoglycemia
What cells secrete ghrelin?	X cells in the body of the stomach

GASTROINTESTINAL CONTROL—MOTILITY

Name the types of electrical waves found in the alimentary tract.	Slow waves and spike potentials
What are slow waves?	Fluctuating changes in the resting membrane potential
What are slow waves *not*?	Action potentials
Where are slow waves generated?	Cells of Cajal (pacemaker of the alimentary tract)
Why are slow waves important?	Determine the rhythmicity of the GI tract's contractions by controlling the pattern of spike potentials
Where in the tract are the waves the slowest?	Stomach at 3 waves/min
Where in the tract are the waves the fastest?	Duodenum at 12 waves/min
What are spike potentials?	Action potentials of the alimentary tract
How are spike potentials generated?	They occur when the resting gut pacemaker membranes depolarize

Name three factors that cause increased depolarization of gut pacemaker cells.

1. Muscle stretch
2. ACh
3. PNS

Which channels are involved in the generation of the action potential?

Ca^{2+}-Na^+ channels, just like anywhere else in the body

How does a spike potential cause contraction?

Like other muscle cells, Ca^{2+} enters the smooth muscle cell interior

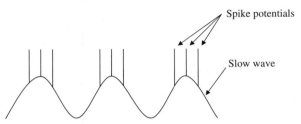

Figure 6.2   Electrical signaling in the GI tract.

Define motility.

Mechanical activity of the GI tract that is divided into mixing (segmentation) and propelling (peristalsis)

Describe segmentation.

Contraction around the bolus sends intestinal contents (chyme) backward and forward. The area then relaxes and the material moves back into the segment, mixing the contents.

Describe peristalsis.

Contraction behind the bolus is coupled with relaxation in front of it, which propels the bolus distally

What factors promote inhibition of peristalsis?

Ileogastric reflex and CCK

Name the functions of small intestinal motility.

Allows for mixing of food bolus with digestive enzymes

Exposes food molecules to absorptive mucosa

Propels nonabsorbed material to the colon

Which aspect of motility is most important in the small intestine?

Segmentation: allows for increased surface area for digestion and absorption of chyme

**What is the frequency of slow waves
in the following segments of the small
intestine?**

    Duodenum

    Proximal jejunum

    Terminal ileum

12 waves/min

12 waves/min

8 to 9 waves/min

**What other factor is important
for segmental contraction?**

Excitation by the myenteric plexus

**What is the average velocity
of peristalsis waves in the small
intestine?**

0.5 to 2.0 cm/s

**What factors stimulate increased
peristalsis activity?**

Gastroileal reflex (neural regulation)

Gastrin

CCK

Serotonin

Insulin

**What factors inhibit peristalsis
activity?**

Secretin and glucagon

**Name the two types of motility found
in the colon.**

1. Haustral segmental movement
2. Mass movement

What are haustra?

Invaginations of the circular and
longitudinal muscles of the large
intestine which provide some
compartmentalization

What are mass movements?

Modified peristalsis that is
characterized by uniform contraction
and movement of colonic contents
down the descending colon

**How often do mass movements occur
per day?**

1 to 3 times/day

**Name some factors that stimulate mass
movement.**

Gastrocolic reflex

Duodenocolic reflex

Irritation of the colon

PNS stimulation

Over distention of a colonic segment

Where is the vomiting center located?

Medulla

What stimuli does the vomiting center respond to?	Gag Gastric distention Vestibular stimulation
Where are the chemoreceptors that can induce vomiting?	Fourth ventricle
What stimuli do the chemoreceptors respond to?	Emetic substances Vestibular stimulation Radiation
What is vomiting?	Reverse peristalsis that propels GI contents in the stomach towards the oropharynx and out through the upper esophageal sphincter
What occurs if the peristalsis is not strong enough to overcome the pressure in the upper esophageal sphincter (UES)?	Retching
Where does the reverse peristalsis begin?	Small intestine

MOUTH AND ESOPHAGUS

Course reduction in food particle size is accomplished by what process?	Mastication
During this process what fluid is introduced to the food bolus?	Saliva
What are the principal glands of salivation?	1. Submandibular (70%) 2. Parotid (25%) 3. Sublingual (5%)
Name the functions of saliva.	Dissolves and alkalinizes ingested food particles Protects the oral cavity Moistens the mouth (lubrication) Begins hydrolysis of complex starches

Name and describe the two types of salivary secretions.

1. Serous secretions: contain enzymes for starch digestion
2. Mucous secretions: contain mucin for lubrication and protection

What is the enzyme found in salivary secretions responsible for carbohydrate digestion?

Salivary amylase

In what ways does saliva help protect the oropharynx?

1. Salivary piece: IgA—binding protein which activates secreted IgA
2. Lactoferrin secretion: chelates iron to make it unavailable for bacteria
3. Lysozyme: attacks bacterial cell walls
4. Acquired pellicle: a thin layer of glycoproteins that adheres to teeth to help protect them

Name the type of secretions for the principal glands:

Parotid

Serous

Submandibular

Serous and mucous

Sublingual

Serous and mucous

Describe the glandular process of saliva secretion:

Initial saliva from gland (isotonic to plasma)
↓
Ducts secrete K^+ and HCO_3^-
↓
Na^+ reabsorption occurs in the salivary ducts in proportion to the time spent there, usually leading to hypotonic saliva

In periods of fasting, when salivary flow is low, how does the composition of saliva change?

The saliva remains in the duct longer and more sodium and chloride are reabsorbed without water, so it becomes hypotonic.

And when salivary flow is rapid?

Quick transit times through the duct leads to secretions that more closely resembles acinar (plasma) composition

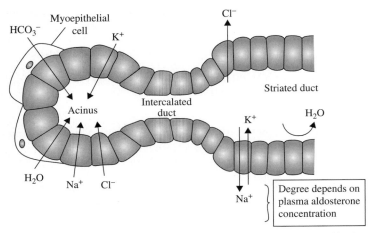

Figure 6.3   The salivary gland. Note that fine tuning of salivary composition is aldosterone responsive.

What regulates saliva production?	PNS and SNS
What effect does the PNS have on saliva production?	Increases it
What effect does the SNS have on saliva production?	Increases it as well
What stimuli increase saliva production?	Presence of food in the mouth Smells Conditioned reflexes (e.g., Pavlov dog) Nausea
What stimuli decrease saliva production?	Dehydration Fear Anticholinergic medications Sleep
Describe swallowing.	A highly coordinated, complicated series of muscular contractions that propels a bolus of food toward the stomach

Where is the swallow center located?	Medulla and lower pons
Which nerves contain the motor impulses from the swallow center?	Cranial nerves (CN) V, IX, X, XII, and the superior CN

Name the stage of the swallow reflex that is described by the following:

Involves voluntary action that squeezes food into the pharynx and against the palate	Voluntary stage (oral)
Involves closure of the trachea, opening of the esophagus, and generation of a peristaltic wave (primary peristalsis) that forces the food bolus into the esophagus	Pharyngeal stage
Involves continuation of primary peristalsis, the relaxation of the upper esophagus, and the entrance of the food bolus into the esophagus	Esophageal stage
How long does it take the primary wave to reach the LES?	5 to 10 seconds (travels at 3-5 cm/s)
When is a secondary peristalsis generated?	When the primary peristalsis wave is insufficient to clear the esophagus of the food bolus
What is receptive relaxation?	A vagovagal reflex that relaxes the LES prior to the peristaltic wave
Why is receptive relaxation important?	Allows for easy propulsion of food bolus into the stomach
What types of secretions are found in the esophagus?	Mucoid
Name its main function.	Provides lubrication for swallowing
What is the mechanism by which gastric contents are able to reflux into the esophagus (e.g., gastroesophageal reflux disease or GERD)?	Decreased LES tone
What can result if the LES tone is increased and it does not relax with swallowing?	Achalasia

STOMACH

Name the five regions of the stomach that are labeled below.

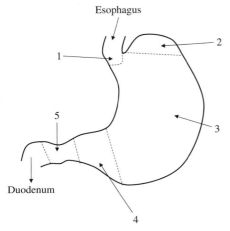

Esophagus

1. Cardia
2. Fundus
3. Body
4. Antrum
5. Pylorus

Duodenum

Figure 6.4   Stomach anatomy.

What are the physiologic divisions of the stomach and what are their boundaries?	Orad portion: extends from the fundus to the proximal body Caudad portion: extends from the distal body to the antrum
What are the three major functions of the stomach?	Store food Make chyme Empty food at a rate suitable for proper digestion and absorption by the small intestine
What is the maximum amount of food that can be stored by the stomach?	1.5 L
What is chyme?	Semifluid paste that results from the food bolus mixing with gastric secretions
What promotes gastric emptying?	Stretch and gastrin
What inhibits gastric emptying?	Increased osmolarity Products of fat digestion pH <3.5

The stomach has five main exocrine secretions. What are they?

Water

Acid

Enzymes (gastrin and pepsin lipase)

Intrinsic factor

Mucus (barrier to protect the mucosa)

Name the cell types with the following description:

Found in the fundus and secretes HCl and intrinsic factor

Parietal cells

Found in the fundus and secretes pepsinogen

Chief cells/peptic cells

Found in antrum and secretes gastrin

G cells

Found in the antrum and secretes mucus and pepsinogen

Mucous cells

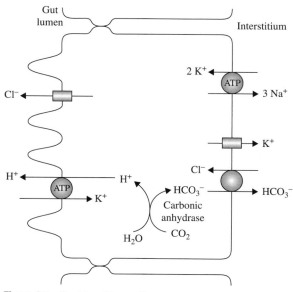

Figure 6.5 Gastric acid secretion.

On the above diagram, can you point out where a proton pump inhibitor would exert its effect?

Luminal H/K ATPase

Name the three factors that work synergistically to promote HCl secretion.

1. Histamine
2. Gastrin
3. Acetylcholine

Name the three different receptors that those factors bind to on parietal cells to stimulate acid secretion.

1. H_2 receptor
2. Gastrin receptor
3. Muscarinic (acetylcholine) receptor

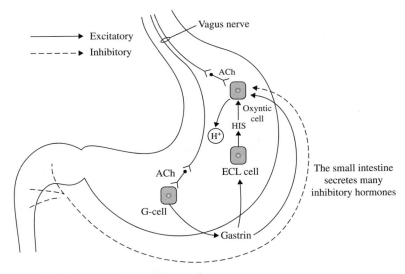

Figure 6.6   Control of gastric acid secretion.

What induces ACh stimulation of H^+ secretion?

Vagus nerve, which directly innervates parietal cells (ACh is the neurotransmitter)

What induces gastrin stimulation of H^+ secretion?

Small peptides present in the lumen

Distension of the stomach

Vagal stimulation (e.g., response to eating)

Name the compounds that can inhibit the following elements of HCl secretion:

ACh

Cholinergic muscarinic antagonists

Histamine

H_2 receptor-blocking agents

Gastrin

None known at this time

Apical H^+-K^+-ATPase

Proton pump inhibitors (PPIs)

Name the phase of gastric secretion that corresponds to the following description:

Occurs before food enters the stomach and results from the sight, smell, and thought of food	Cephalic phase
Mediated entirely by vagal impulses and accounts for 20% to 30% of the total gastric secretion	Cephalic phase
Begins when stomach is distended by food	Gastric phase
Mediated by vagovagal reflex, enteric reflexes, and gastrin	Gastric phase
Accounting for > 70% of the total gastric secretion	Gastric phase

What phase begins when food arrives in the duodenum?

Intestinal phase

What is the precursor to pepsin?

Pepsinogen

What cells secrete pepsinogen?

Chief cells

What activates pepsinogen?

pH below 5; once activated it can also autocatalyze the formation of additional pepsin

What is the role of pepsin in digestion?

It cleaves the peptide bonds found in protein products

What protein, secreted by parietal cells, is later reabsorbed in the terminal ileum?

Intrinsic factor

What is the function of intrinsic factor?

To bind vitamin B_{12} for absorption in the small intestine

How does the gastric mucosa protect itself from the hostile acidity of the gastric lumen?

A layer of secreted mucus serves as a barrier. HCO_3^- that is secreted gets trapped in the glycoproteins as well. The oxyntic (chief) cells also have a thick plasma membrane and tight junctions between them that prevent back diffusion of H^+.

What is an important stimulus for secretion of the mucus barrier?

Prostaglandins

ACCESSORY DIGESTIVE ORGANS

What three organs are considered the accessory digestive organs?

1. The exocrine pancreas
2. Liver
3. Gall bladder

What is the primary function of the pancreas?

To add additional digestive enzymes and an alkaline solution to the digestive chyme in the small bowel

Why is the alkaline fluid important?

Two reasons: firstly, the acidic chyme would be caustic to the poorly defended bowel, and secondly, the pancreatic enzymes have optimum activity at a neutral pH

Name the three types of cells found in the pancreas.

1. Acinar cells
2. Islet cells (see Chapter 7)
3. Duct cells

What is the structure of the pancreatic exocrine glands?

It is very similar to that of the salivary glands. It has a central acini connected to a series of ducts that deliver its products to the bowel lumen.

How do ductal cells modify pancreatic secretions?

They secrete bicarbonate and reabsorb potassium

How does secretory rate influence the composition of pancreatic juice?

Rapid flow rates reduce the transit time through the ducts and so the ductal cells are less able to modify the secretions leading to less alkalinity and more K^+ secretion

How does the endocrine pancreas relate to the exocrine pancreas?

The islet cells lie cradled between the pancreatic acini with a rich vascular supply but they have no continuity with the exocrine ducts.

For the following secretion, name its cell of origin:

Zymogens (proteolytic enzymes)   Acinar cells

Glucagon   Islet cells (alpha cells)

Insulin   Islet cells (beta cells)

Somatostatin   Islet cells (delta cells)

Isosmotic sodium bicarbonate solution   Duct cells

What is a zymogen?	It is a proteolytic precursor. In this form, these enzymes are inactive.
Where are they activated?	In the bowel lumen by trypsinogen which is activated by enterokinase, a brush border enzyme
Why is the activation of these enzymes so tightly regulated?	If they were activated in the pancreas, autodigestion would occur.

Name the enzyme with the following catalytic function:

Cleaves peptide bonds adjacent to basic amino acids	Trypsin
Cleaves peptide bonds adjacent to aromatic amino acids	Chymotrypsin
Cleaves carboxy terminal amino acids with aromatic or branched side chains	Carboxy peptidase A
Cleaves carboxy terminal amino acids with basic side chains	Carboxy peptidase B
Cleaves bonds in elastin	Elastase
Cleaves phospholipid to fatty acids and lysophospholipids	Phospholipase A
Hydrolyzes starches, glycogen, and other carbohydrates	Amylase

What substances stimulate the acinar cells?	Acetylcholine and CCK
Which substances stimulate the ductal cells?	Secretin
What is the primary digestive function of the liver?	To produce and secrete bile
What are the other functions of the liver?	Carbohydrate metabolism
	Cholesterol metabolism
	Fat metabolism
	Amino acid and protein synthesis
	Storage of fat soluble vitamins, vitamin $B_{12,}$ iron and copper
	Immune functions
	Detoxification and biotransformation
What are the structural units of the liver?	Liver lobules

What are the functional units of the liver?	Liver acinus
How are these liver acini defined?	They are a collection of hepatocytes that receive a blood supply from the same arteriole and are drained by the same venule
What is unique about the liver's blood supply?	It receives some oxygenated blood and some deoxygenated blood. The oxygenated blood coming from the hepatic artery off of the celiac axis, and the deoxygenated component coming from the portal circulation.
When discussing single liver acini, what is meant by "Zone III"?	Since the liver receives relatively low oxygen volumes, the hepatocytes nearest the arteriole tend to have different cellular apparatus than those further away. The hepatocytes nearest the arteriole fall into Zone I, and the hepatocytes around the central vein are within Zone III.
Which zone tends to undertake oxidative reactions, as well as bile acid production reactions?	Zone I
What types of reactions occur in Zone III?	Ketogenesis, glycolysis, etc (those requiring low oxygen tension)
Where is bile stored?	Gallbladder
Name the three main functions of bile.	1. Helps with fat digestion and absorption 2. Helps excrete waste products such as bilirubin 3. Assists in neutralizing the gastric contents
Name the main components of bile.	1. Bile salts 2. Lecithin 3. Bilirubin 4. Cholesterol
What are bile acids?	Amphipathic molecules that have a hydrophobic tail attached to several polar groups
What are bile salts?	Bile acids conjugated to amino acids: glycine and taurine (i.e., taurocholic)

What do bile acids do with respect to fat absorption?

When released as bile salts into the gut, some of them dissociate into their bile acid forms. These molecules then coalesce with lecithin into micelles which provide a hydrophobic environment for cholesterols, fats (especially long chain fatty acids), and other hydrophobic molecules to dissolve in.

Where is bile stored?

In the gallbladder

What is meant by the term "enterohepatic circulation?"

This describes a process by which bile acids are secreted into the gut for elimination, but then are reabsorbed and returned to the liver by the portal circulation

Why is this particularly important when discussing bile acids?

The bile acid pool is not large enough to allow for absorption of the fat in a normal meal; as such, the bile salts are recycled and secreted back into the gut.

What is bilirubin?

A product of hemoglobin destruction

What is unconjugated bilirubin?

When senescent RBCs are broken down the free bilirubin circulates loosely bound to albumin, this is a measure of the quantity of bilirubin in that state

What happens to unconjugated bilirubin?

It is then taken up by hepatocytes where the enzyme glucuronyl transferase conjugates the bilirubin

Once it is secreted in bile, what two routes can conjugated bilirubin take to be excreted?

1. It can be secreted in the feces unaltered
2. It can be metabolized by bacteria in the gut to urobilinogen which can then be either excreted in the feces or it can be reabsorbed and then secreted in the kidney

What is jaundice?

The yellowing of skin

How does jaundice develop?

Through the increase in total body bilirubin. This can happen by:
1. Excess production (i.e., increased RBC breakdown), this is considered *prehepatic* jaundice
2. Excretory failure, this is either *hepatic or posthepatic* jaundice(i.e., liver failure, or obstruction, respectively)

The gallbladder stores bile salts in a dehydrated form; what is the stimulus for release of bile?

1. CCK during the intestinal phase (strongest stimuli)
2. Vagal input during the cephalic phase
3. Fatty food in the duodenum

Name the three stimuli that relax the sphincter of Oddi.

1. Peristaltic waves of the intestine (strongest stimuli)
2. Contraction of gallbladder
3. CCK

SMALL BOWEL—GENERAL THROUGH DIGESTION

The small intestine is divided into what three anatomic regions?

Duodenum, jejunum, and ileum

What is the primary feature of the small bowel that makes it ideal for digestion and absorption?

Massive surface area

What are the three anatomic features to the small intestine that increases its absorption capacity 1000-fold?

Valvulae conniventes (folds of Kerckring)
Villi
Microvilli

What is the functional unit of the small intestine called?

The villus

What are the three divisions of an intestinal villus?

1. The villus tip
2. The maturation zone
3. The crypt

What happens in the crypt?

Stem cells are continually dividing to replenish sloughed off enterocytes

In which zone do cells begin to express secretory qualities?

The maturation zone

How long does a fully-developed enterocyte remain at the villus tip?

Usually only 3 to 4 days

Does small (and large) bowel mucosa *secrete* fluid into the bowel lumen?

Yes; while the villus tip cells are proficient at reabsorption, the crypt cells tend to be secretors

When does this secretory mechanism become clinically significant?

When there is injury to the villi; the crypt continues to secrete contributing to diarrhea and electrolyte loss

Besides offering a huge surface area for absorption, what is the other key role the small intestine plays in digestion?	It is the site where most of the digestive enzymes which break down food are found
What is the difference in the three types of digestion listed below?	
Luminal digestion	This occurs within the lumen, catalyzed by secreted enzymes
Membrane digestion	This is mediated by the action of enzymes that are fixed to the brush border of enterocytes
Intracellular digestion	This is mediated by enzymes that are in the cytoplasm of enterocytes or in organelles, materials must be absorbed for this type of digestion to occur.
Name three major sources of carbohydrate in the diet.	1. Starch 2. Sucrose 3. Lactose
What is the final product of carbohydrate digestion?	Monosaccharides
Name the major monosaccharides.	1. Glucose (80%) 2. Galactose 3. Fructose
Name the location where the following enzymes can be found:	
α-Dextrinase	Intestinal brush border
Isomaltase/sucrase	Intestinal brush border
Lactase	Intestinal brush border
Maltase	Intestinal brush border
Ptyalin (alpha-amylase)	Saliva
Pancreatic amylase	Pancreatic secretions
Trehalase	Intestinal brush border
Name the enzyme used to digest the following:	
Starch	Ptyalin and pancreatic amylase
Lactose	Lactase
Sucrose	Sucrase
Maltose	Maltase
Alpha-limit dextrin	α-Dextrinase

Name the sources of proteins targeted for digestion.	1. Dietary protein 2. Tissue protein 3. Sloughed cells of GI tract 4. Pancreatic secretions

Name the location for the following enzymes of protein digestion:

Carboxy polypeptidase	Pancreatic secretions
Chymotrypsin	Pancreatic secretions
Pepsin	Stomach
Peptidases	Intestinal brush border
Proelastase	Intestinal brush border
Trypsin	Pancreatic secretions

What are the final products of protein digestion?	1. Amino acids (99%) 2. Dipeptides/tripeptides (<1%)
What *fats* are found in the diet?	Triglycerides Cholesterol esters Phospholipids Cholesterol Fat-soluble vitamins (A, D, E, and K)
Which fat is the most abundant?	Triglycerides
Where is the main site of fat digestion?	Small intestine
What makes fat digestion different from the digestion of carbohydrates and proteins?	The need for emulsification
Why is emulsification important?	Increases surface area for which digestive enzymes can operate
What is required for emulsification?	Bile salts and lecithin to form micelles
Why are micelles important in digestion?	As mentioned during our bile discussion, they provide a hydrophobic carrier for absorptive purposes

Name the enzyme used to digest the following:

Triglycerides	Pancreatic lipase
Cholesterol ester	Cholesterol esterase
Phospholipid	Phospholipase A2

Name the end product of digestion for the following:

Triglycerides	Free fatty acids and two monoglycerides
Cholesterol ester	Free fatty acid and cholesterol
Phospholipid	Free fatty acid and lysophospholipid

SMALL BOWEL—ABSORPTION

The basic mechanisms of absorption are:
1. Solvent drag
2. Passive diffusion
3. Facilitated diffusion
4. Active transport

What is the main mechanism used to absorb water?

Diffusion

How much water is absorbed per day?

Between 5 L and 10 L

What is the average rate of water absorption by the small intestine?

200 to 400 mL/h

Name the mechanisms used to absorb sodium.

Simple diffusion

Facilitated diffusion

Solvent drag

Primary active transport

Secondary active transport

Which is the most important mechanism for sodium absorption?

Secondary active transport, aka, Cotransport with other solutes who use the sodium gradient generated by the basolateral ATPase to enter enterocytes

Give examples of nutrients coupled to sodium's absorption.

Chloride, amino acids, and glucose

Name the potent stimuli for sodium's absorption.

Aldosterone

Name the mechanism(s) used for chloride's absorption.

Passive diffusion and exchange for HCO_3^-

What is the primary mechanism of water reabsorption in the small intestine?

Isosmotic transport; water follows absorption of nutrients and electrolytes. Bear in mind though, that a chyme bolus is often hypertonic and early in the small bowel water flows *into* the bowel before being recovered later.

Briefly discuss carbohydrate absorption from the gut lumen (be sure to include necessary substrate as well as transport mechanisms).

As mentioned above, digestion must reduce carbohydrates to monosaccharides for absorption in the small intestine. This happens relatively early in the small bowel and *most* of the monosaccharides have been absorbed by the time chime reaches the jejunum. The transporters used are primarily SGLT 1, and GLUT 5 (see Fig. 6.7). SGLT 1 is important because it is a sodium-dependent cotransporter (an example of facilitated diffusion).

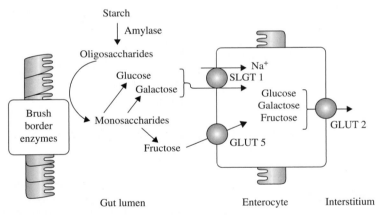

Figure 6.7   Carbohydrate digestion and absorption.

Describe the process of glucose and galactose absorption.

Active transport of sodium across the basolateral membrane by Na^+-K^+-ATPase creates a Na^+ concentration gradient across the apical membrane. An apical membrane cotransport protein couples the influx of Na^+ and sugar affectively driving sugar into the cell (secondary active t-port).

Name the other glucose transport mechanism.

Solvent drag (at high concentrations of glucose) and facilitated diffusion through the basolateral membrane

How is fructose absorbed?

Facilitated diffusion utilizing sodium-independent insulin-independent transporter (GLUT 5)

What transporter delivers all monosaccharides from the enterocyte to the adjacent capillary?

GLUT 2

Protein digestion results in both peptide and single amino acid products, how are each absorbed?

Some of the resultant peptides are brought into enterocytes by a H^+ coupled mechanism where they are broken into single amino acids; most, though, are hydrolyzed to single amino acids before they are absorbed by cotransport

Where are most protein peptides absorbed?

Through the luminal membranes of the intestinal epithelial cells

How are most single amino acids absorbed?

Sodium-dependent cotransporter system

Where in the GI tract are most fats absorbed?

Jejunum

Which fatty acids can move freely through luminal membranes after digestion?

Short and medium chain fatty acids only

With appropriate bile acid production and secretion, how much dietary fat is absorbed?

97%

If bile acid production/secretion is impaired, how much dietary fat is absorbed?

40% to 50%

What are chylomicrons?

Globules of reformed/repackaged triglycerides, cholesterol, and phospholipids that are arranged in a manner similar to micelles

What is the role of chylomicron formation?	Allows for systemic transport of fat via exocytosis
What is essential for the exocytosis of chylomicrons?	Apoprotein B: helps the chylomicron attach to cell membrane before it is expelled
Are chylomicrons delivered directly to the adjacent capillaries?	No, they are delivered to the lymphatics of the gut, transported through the lymphatic system and finally dumped into the blood stream centrally (into the left brachiocephalic vein)
What happens to these chylomicrons?	They are transported to the skeletal muscle cells and adipose tissue expressing lipoprotein lipase where they are used/stored. Whatever is not taken up there is transported to the liver where it is repackaged.
What are the fat-soluble vitamins?	Vitamins A, D, E, and K
What is unique about vitamin B_{12} absorption?	It requires intrinsic factor (IF)
Where is vitamin B_{12} absorbed?	Terminal ileum
What results when there is a lack of IF?	Pernicious anemia (a megaloblastic anemia common in the elderly and those with a predisposition for autoimmune disease)
Where is vitamin B_{12} stored in the body?	In the liver
How long can we rely on those stores?	2 to 3 months
How are water soluble vitamins absorbed?	Both by simple diffusion as well as by cotransport and countertransport
Using Table 6.1, consider the various vitamins. Name their functions as well as what you might expect to find if a patient is deficient in them.	

Table 6.1 Vitamins

Vitamin	Function	Deficiency
A (β-carotene)	Pigment in retina	Night blindness Hyperkeratosis
B$_1$ (thiamine)	Coenzyme in pyruvate and α-ketoacid metabolism	Beriberi
B$_2$ (riboflavin)	Coenzyme in mitochondrial oxidative metabolism	Normocytic anemia
B$_3$ (niacin)	Coenzyme in mitochondrial oxidative metabolism	Pellagra
B$_6$ (pyridoxine)	Coenzyme in amino acid synthesis	Normocytic anemia
B$_{12}$ (cobalamin)	Facilitates formation of erythrocytes and neuronal myelin sheath	Pernicious anemia
C (ascorbic acid)	Coenzyme in hydroxyproline formation, used in collagen	Scurvy
D (cholecalciferol)	Increased Ca^{2+} absorption	Rickets (childhood deficiency)
E (α-tocopherol)	Antioxidant	Peripheral neuropathy
K$_1$ (phylloquinone)	Blood clotting: needed for synthesis of factors VII, IX, X, and prothrombin	Hemorrhage
Folate	Purine synthesis	Megaloblastic anemia
Biotin	Coenzyme for carboxylation reactions	Neurologic signs
Pantothenic acid	Coenzyme A: needed for metabolism of carbohydrate and fat via acetyl-coenzyme A and amino acid synthesis	Neurologic and gastrointestinal signs

(Reproduced, with permission, from Kibble JD, Halsey CR: *Medical Physiology: The Big Picture.* New York, NY: McGraw-Hill; 2009.)

LARGE BOWEL AND DEFECATION

Where, anatomically, is the ileocecal valve?	Between the ileum and the cecum, usually in the right lower quadrant
What is the principal function of the ileocecal valve?	Prevents backflow of colonic contents into the small intestine
Why is prevention of reflux important?	The colons motility involves the shuffling of large amounts of chyme forward and backward as it tries to extract the last of the usable electrolytes and water; there is also a large volume of bacteria that reside in the gut that we do not want in our small bowel.
How long does it take to move chyme from the ileocecal valve to the transverse colon?	8 to 15 hours
What is significant about the gut flora of the colon?	The resident flora provide some of the final modifications to the chyme helping to liberate the last of the usable elements from our diets
What vitamin depends on gut bacteria for production?	Vitamin K; this is why we give infants, who don't yet have gut flora, an injection of vitamin K at birth
What is the mechanism for water resorption in the proximal colon?	Water follows Na^+ reabsorption mediated by an apical membrane Na^+/H^+ exchanger
What is the mechanism for water resorption in the distal colon?	A Na^+-K^+ exchange system that resembles the one used in the distal tubule of the kidney; in fact, it too is responsive to aldosterone, but its overall impact on systemic Na^+ concentration is far weaker
What initiates the desire for defecation?	Presence of feces in the rectum

Name the defecation reflex described
by the following:

Uses enteric nervous system to initiate peristaltic waves in the descending colon, sigmoid, and rectum, thus forcing feces toward the anus	Intrinsic colonic reflex
Uses parasympathetic fibers in the pelvic nerves to intensify the peristaltic wave, relax the internal anal sphincter, and converts the intrinsic defecation reflex into a powerful process	Parasympathetic defecation reflex, coordination of this reflex is trained in youngsters

CLINICAL VIGNETTES

A patient goes to his doctor complaining of reflux. The patient undergoes an extensive workup that finds a decrease in pH of the stomach and hypertrophy and hyperplasia of the gastric mucosa. The patient is diagnosed with a tumor that secretes a certain hormone. What hormone is it secreting?

Gastrin. The actions of gastrin are to increase H^+ secretion by the gastric parietal cells and to stimulate the growth of the gastric mucosa.

In order to isolate gastrin from the human bloodstream, a researcher has designed a radioactive probe that is specific to the last five amino acids on the C-terminal of the protein. During the purification of the protein, he finds that he continues to have two different proteins. What is the other protein that the researcher is purifying?

Cholecystokinin (CCK). The structure of the five C-terminal amino acids are identical to those of gastrin.

The following mixtures are ingested by a volunteer:

Mixture 1: Small peptide and amino acids

Mixture 2: Fatty acids

Mixture 3: Triglycerides

After each mixture, the patient's level of CCK is measured. Which mixture will have no affect on CCK levels?

Mixture 3, since triglycerides do not cross the intestinal cell membranes

A researcher studying somatostatin has designed an experiment in which he has injected a volunteer with this hormone and then measured the relative levels of each gastrointestinal (GI) hormone pre- and postinjection. For each of the following hormones, indicate the affect (either ↑/↓) of somatostatin on its level: gastrin, CCK, secretin, and gastric inhibitory peptide (GIP).

All ↓. Somatostatin inhibits the release of all of the GI hormones and also inhibits gastric hydrogen ion secretion. Clinically, somatostatin (Octreotide) is used to shut down GI function and help to reduce blood flow to the region when patients are experiencing GI bleeding.

A 35-year-old woman has come to her doctor with the complaint of watery diarrhea and flushing for the past year. She says that she has over 10 watery stools per day and is concerned because it is starting to hinder her abilities at work. Upon further questioning, the woman also expresses concern over pain in the upper abdomen that radiates to the back. Blood analysis shows hyperglycemia, hypercalcemia, and hypokalemia. A hormone-secreting tumor is found to be the cause of this patient's symptoms. What hormone is it secreting?

VIP. This tumor is known as a VIPoma. VIP is a potent stimulator of cyclic adenosine monophosphate (cAMP) production in the gut, which leads to massive secretion of water and electrolyte (mainly potassium). They can be associated with multiple endocrine neoplasia (MEN) I syndrome.

A 3-day-old boy is being evaluated in the newborn nursery because he has clear abdominal distension and has yet to pass meconium. Following a complete examination, a digital rectal examination is done followed by a voluminous passage of meconium. What is the most likely explanation?

This youngster likely has Hirschsprung disease, which develops from failure of neural crest cells to appropriately migrate to the distal colon. This leads to an absence of the myenteric plexus and, therefore, failure of colonic motility. The aganglionic segment fails to relax and the normally innervated proximal bowel dilates. Stool fails to pass because of the strong distal contraction.

A 2-year-old male is brought to your office with complaints of persistent voluminous diarrhea. Mom tells you that it has been going on for several months, and she is worried about how this is impacting his growth and development. Upon further questioning, you realize that this started within a week or two of the introduction of cereals into his diet.

What is the most likely diagnosis?

Celiac sprue; other typical symptoms include bloating, flatulence, and steatorrhea.

What is the pathophysiology?

Immunologic dysfunction leads to the destruction of intestinal villi. This leads to poor nutrient absorption as well as poor water reclamation.

What do you tell mom about growth and development?

It can lead to growth problems due to lack of growth substrate and vitamin deficiencies. In this boy's case, though, with dietary changes (withholding gluten based products), he should be able to bounce back.

A researcher is studying the effects of flow of saliva and its electrolyte concentrations. For each of the electrolytes, the researcher measured its value when it is initially secreted from the acinus and when it is secreted from the salivary duct. He took measurements at high and low saliva flow rate and then compared them. What should the results look like? Use the chart below to show whether the respective electrolyte is at its highest or lowest concentration, respectively.

Low Flow	High Flow
Na^+	
K^+	
Cl^-	
HCO_3^-	

	Low flow	High flow
Na^+	Lowest	Highest
K^+	Highest	Lowest
Cl^-	Lowest	Highest
HCO_3^-	Unchanged	Unchanged

The salivary ducts reabsorb Na^+ and Cl^-, while it secretes K^+. So the longer it stays in the salivary duct the more Na^+ and Cl^- is reabsorbed and more K^+ is secreted into the saliva. HCO_3^- is the only one that does not follow this rule and it is continuously excreted.

The same researcher decides that he is going to study the pancreas now. But now he wants to know the relative concentration of the electrolytes compared to blood at high flow of pancreatic secretions. Indicate whether the concentration of electrolyte is higher or lower to that of the blood at high flow of pancreatic secretions?

Relative concentration compared to blood
Na^+
K^+
Cl^-
HCO_3^-

Relative concentration compared to blood	
Na^+	Same
K^+	Same
Cl^-	Lower
HCO_3^-	Higher

At high flow, the pancreas secretes a fluid that is mostly Na^+ and HCO_3^-. At low flow, the pancreas secrets mostly Na^+ and Cl^-.

A new device has been invented that measures contraction of the gallbladder. After injection of substance X, the device shows a powerful contraction of the gallbladder. What GI hormone would cause this action?

CCK. Not only does it cause the contraction of the gallbladder, but it also leads to relaxation of the sphincter of Oddi to facilitate bile entry into the duodenum.

A strange poison has been found that only inhibits the Na$^+$-K$^+$ ATP-ase in the basolateral membrane of the GI tract. What affect does this have on the absorption of glucose and galactose?

Glucose and galactose are absorbed through the Na$^+$-dependent cotransporter in the luminal membrane. If the Na$^+$-K$^+$ pump is inhibited, then the Na$^+$ gradient is lessened, leading to inhibition of glucose and galactose absorption.

***Vibrio cholerae* causes diarrhea by secreting a toxin that activates adenylate cyclase, which leads to increase of cAMP. Why does this lead to diarrhea?**

The increased intracellular cAMP results in opening of the Cl$^-$ channels in the luminal membrane. The flow of Cl$^-$ out of the cell into the GI tract "traps" Na$^+$ in the gut lumen, thereby trapping H$_2$O. This leads to a secretory diarrhea.

A researcher is studying the sympathetic stimulation during a stressful situation. For the following GI tract activities, indicate the expected response:

Digestion	Lowers digestion
Secretion	Lowers secretion
Motor activity	Lowers motor activity

Consider the role of the sympathetic nervous system on gut motility. Note that some people, most talked-about being those with irritable bowel syndrome, respond differently, the reasons for this have not yet been fully elucidated.

A patient is given an injection of a vitamin and then is told to swallow a pill containing the same vitamin tagged with a radioactive substance. Twenty-four hours later, the patient's urine is negative for the radioactive vitamin. Name the above test and its purpose.

Schilling test. It is conducted to determine the etiology of vitamin B$_{12}$ deficiency. In the given example, the parenteral B$_{12}$ saturates the circulating storage pools, the oral B$_{12}$ challenges the physiologic route of absorption. Subsequent lack of tagged vitamin B$_{12}$ in urine suggests lack of B$_{12}$ absorption, probably due to a lack of intrinsic factor (IF).

A researcher is studying the sequela of fat-soluble vitamin deficiency. For each description below, identify the deficient vitamin.

Night blindness and dry skin	Vitamin A
Bendable bones in children	Vitamin D
Hypoprothrombinemia	Vitamin K
Increased fragility of RBCs	Vitamin E

A 17-year-old female presents to her primary care doctor with a 7-month history of intermittent diarrhea with light colored, sticky stools (evidence of increasing fat in her stool), gum bleeding, and abdominal bloating. After extensive workup, she was diagnosed with celiac disease. Explain her symptoms.

In certain hosts, gliadin antigens can, for some reason, lead to sensitization of T cells to additional gliadin exposure. Further exposure to gliadin (one of the protein constituents of gluten) leads to immune activation and progressive bowel injury. In these susceptible people, the villi are lost and the surface epithelium of the gut is immature. This leads to loss of absorptive surface, deficiency of mucosal enzymes. In this young woman she has suffered from bowel inflammation for a long time, her bowel tends to be predominately secretory with consequent diarrhea, the loss of absorptive mucosa leads to fat malabsorption, and with all of this vitamin deficiency is common, in her case we see the effects of vitamin K deficiency (and resultant deficiency of the vitamin K dependent coagulation proteins) as gum bleeding.

A 54-year-old woman comes into your office complaining of epigastric pain of 5 months' duration. It began as intermittent pain, but has become more painful in recent weeks. On further questioning you discover she has been using the maximum daily dose of aspirin to help with joint pain. What is going on?

The aspirin is likely inhibiting the prostaglandin production in the gastric mucosa. As a consequence the mucosa sees less stimuli for mucus secretion and the stomach has far less protection from its own acid. This condition is called erosive gastritis and is extremely common in clinical practice.

A 7-year-old female immigrant from Argentina presents with progressing difficulty in swallowing food. You diagnose her with *Trypanosoma cruzi* infection, and determine that the myenteric plexi of her esophagus has been attacked? What does this lead to clinically?

Achalasia. In patients from South or Central America exposed to possible *Trypanosoma cruzi* infection, clinicians should be attentive to this disease. The loss of esophageal neurons leads progressive peristaltic dysfunction and failure of the lower esophageal sphincter to relax allowing passage of food into the stomach. Esophageal dilation results, called Chagas' disease.

A 19-year-old female is brought by her mom to emergency department (ED) due to bizarre behavior and dysarthria. Workup revealed decreased ceruloplasmin. She was subsequently diagnosed with Wilson disease. What is ceruloplasmin and why is it elevated in Wilson disease?

Ceruloplasmin is the carrier protein for copper in the body. In Wilson disease copper metabolism is dysfunctional which leads to inadequate incorporation of copper into apoceruloplasmin (once it binds copper $\rightarrow$ ceruloplasmin). Apoceruloplasmin is rapidly degraded in the blood leading to low total ceruloplasmin levels.

Copper largely accumulates in the liver, but the copper that does circulate is deposited in various tissues including the brain, the heart, and the iris leading to the prototypical clinical presentation.

A 30-year-old male presents with halitosis, difficulty initiating swallow and regurgitation of food days after ingestion. What is causing his presentation and where is it located?

Zenker diverticulum. It is an outpouching that results from a defect in the cricopharyngeal muscle. This is the prototypical presentation, although usually it occurs in older individuals.

CHAPTER 7

Endocrine Physiology

HORMONES

What is a hormone?

A chemical substance, formed in a tissue or organ and carried in the blood, that stimulates or inhibits the growth or function of one or more other tissues or organs

What is an endocrine pathway?

A hormone secreted into blood that acts on distant target cells

What is a paracrine pathway?

A hormone released from one cell that acts on neighboring cells

What is an autocrine pathway?

A hormone released that acts on the cell that secreted it

What is the fundamental mechanism of all hormone action?

Reversible, noncovalent binding to specific receptors on or in target cell

What are the three major classes of hormones?

1. Peptide hormones
2. Steroid hormones
3. Amine hormones

How are polypeptide hormones synthesized?

Peptide hormones are produced en masse during times of quiet and subsequently released into circulation in response to stimuli

Preprohormone produced
from mRNA
↓ proteins cleaved
Prohormone
↓ cleaved
Hormone (Golgi apparatus)
↓
Packaged into secretory
granules for release

199

How are steroid hormones synthesized?

Steroid hormones are not stored in intracellular vesicles and must be synthesized on demand. They use the following general pathway:

Cholesterol
↓
Pregnenolone (mitochondria)
↓
Side chain modifications
(in the endoplasmic reticulum)
↓
Various hormones

How are amino acid hormones synthesized?

Production is similar to peptide hormones in that they are synthesized and stored, but tend to be smaller, generally simpler, molecules

Tyrosine
↓ hydroxylation
↓ decarboxylation
Dopamine
↓ (many steps)
Various hormones

Where are polypeptide hormone receptors?

On the surface of target cell membranes

Where are steroid hormone receptors?

In the target cell cytoplasm

Where are amino acid hormone receptors?

These can be either on or inside the target cells. Two examples are:

Catecholamines: on target cell membrane

Thyroid hormones: in target cell cytoplasm

From Chap. 2, what is meant by "second messenger cascade"?

These are the systems that are used by receptors (of various types) that utilize intermediaries to cause intracellular changes

What are G-proteins?

A second messenger system; guanosine 5'-triphosphate (GTP)-binding proteins that couple hormone receptors on the cell surface to a secondary messenger system inside the cell

What type of intrinsic property do G-proteins have?   GTPase activity

What types of G-proteins are there?   Either stimulatory (G_s) or inhibitory (G_i)

What are G-proteins comprised of and what determines activity?   Three subunits: alpha, beta, and gamma. When the alpha subunit is bound to GTP, the G-protein is activated. It is inactivated when bound to GDP.

Describe, in words, the mechanism of the cyclic adenosine monophosphate (cAMP) second messenger system.

Hormone binds G-protein-coupled receptor on membrane
↓
GDP replaced by GTP to activate G-protein
↓
Activation of adenylate cyclase
↓
↑ $[cAMP]_{intracellular}$
↓
↑ protein kinase A phosphorylation of proteins
↓
Activation/inhibition of a metabolic process

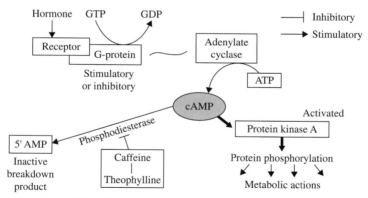

Figure 7.1   cAMP pathway. Note that caffeine and theophylline both inhibit phosphodiesterase, thereby maintaining cAMP as active.

Describe, in words, the mechanism of the inositol triphosphate (IP$_3$) second messenger system.

Hormone binds G-protein-coupled receptor
↓
Activates phospholipase C
↓
Frees diacylglycerol (DAG) + IP$_3$ from membrane
↓
Ca^{2+} release from ER
↓
Activates protein kinase C
↓
phosphorylation of proteins
↓
Activation/inhibition of a metabolic process

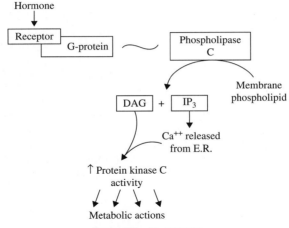

Figure 7.2   IP$_3$ pathway.

Describe, in words, the mechanism of the intracellular Ca^{2+}-calmodulin second messenger system.

Hormone binds G-protein-coupled receptor
↓
Activates membrane Ca^{2+} channel and also releases Ca^{2+} from ER
↓
↑ intracellular Ca^{2+}
↓
↑ Ca^{2+}-calmodulin complex
↓
Regulation of other enzyme activities

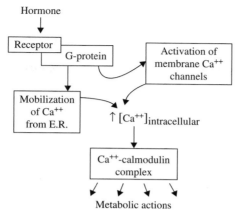

Figure 7.3 Ca^{2+}-calmodulin pathway.

Describe the mechanism of the steroid hormone activation.

Steroid hormone crosses cell membrane (readily soluble in lipid bilayer)
↓
Binds to cytoplasmic receptor
↓
Hormone-receptor complex enters nucleus
↓
Exposes DNA-binding domain on receptor
↓
Complex interacts with DNA to initiate or upregulate transcription
↓
Protein is then synthesized which activates physiologic pathways

What are the two principles of hormone receptor reregulation?

1. Down-regulation: ↓ number or affinity of receptor for a hormone
2. Up-regulation: ↑ number or affinity of a receptor for a hormone

Generally speaking, why does reregulation occur?

It occurs in response to over- or understimulation. An overstimulated receptor will be down regulated to limit activation and vice versa.

What are the two principles of regulation of hormone secretion?

1. Negative feedback (most common)
2. Positive feedback (rare)

What is negative feedback?

A hormone's actions directly or indirectly inhibit its own secretion—a self-terminating cycle

What is positive feedback?

A hormone's actions directly or indirectly promote its own secretion—a self-perpetuating cycle. These cycles are far rarer than negative feedback cycles.

HYPOTHALAMUS AND PITUITARY GLAND

Name the hormones of the:

Anterior pituitary

Thyroid stimulating hormone (TSH)
Luteinizing hormone (LH)
Follicle stimulating hormone (FSH)
Growth hormone (GH)
Prolactin (PRL)
Adrenocorticotropic hormone (ACTH)

Posterior pituitary

Oxytocin
Antidiuretic hormone (ADH)

The following hormones are released from the hypothalamus, name the corresponding pituitary hormones and their respective functions:

Thyrotropin-releasing hormone (TRH)

↑ TSH, PRL secretion; encourages thyroid synthesis and secretion, as well as prolactin secretion

Gonadotropin-releasing hormone (GnRH)

↑ LH, FSH secretion; important regulatory elements of the sex hormones

Corticotropin-releasing hormone (CRH)

↑ ACTH secretion (and α-[MSH], β-endorphin); stimulates the adrenal cortex to release cortisol

Growth hormone-releasing hormone (GHRH)

↑ GH secretion; a complex hormone that influences catabolism throughout the body.

Somatostatin (SS)

↓ release of GH, TSH (among others); a counterregulatory hormone

Prolactin inhibitory factor (PIF)

↓ release of prolactin; another regulatory hormone

Name the anatomic connection between the hypothalamus and the following:

Anterior pituitary

Hypothalamic-hypophysial portal system

Posterior pituitary

Hypothalamic tract

What is unique about the posterior lobe?

It is a collection of nerve axons whose cell bodies are located within the hypothalamus

What is the hypothalamic-hypophysial portal system?

Capillaries that carry blood from the hypothalamus to the anterior pituitary and from the anterior pituitary back to the hypothalamus

What is meant by retrograde blood flow in the hypophysial portal system?

Blood flow traveling from the pituitary back to the hypothalamus

What is the significance of the retrograde blood flow?

Feedback to the hypothalamus

How are the anterior pituitary hormones categorized?

GH-related hormones

Glycoprotein hormones

Corticotropin-related hormones

What is unique about the homology of the following?

GH-related hormones

GH is a polypeptide and is homologous with PRL and HPL

Glycoprotein hormones

All contain α- and β-subunits—α-subunits are similar; hormonal activity comes from β-subunits

Corticotropin related hormones

All are from the same precursor, proopiomelanocortin (POMC)

Describe the POMC protein.

It is a long protein that can be variably cleaved into different proteins, depending on the stage of development and the needs of the organism

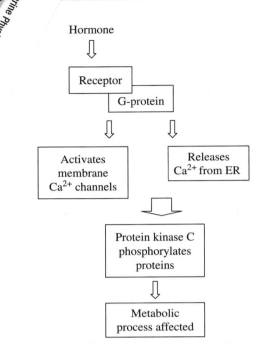

Hormone

⇩

Receptor

G-protein

⇩   ⇩

| Activates membrane Ca^{2+} channels | Releases Ca^{2+} from ER |

⇩

Protein kinase C phosphorylates proteins

⇩

Metabolic process affected

Figure 7.4   POMC processing. The portion of POMC that is cleaved determines the metabolic activity.

Name the actions of the anterior pituitary hormones.

TSH	↑ T_3 and T_4 production (see thyroid section)
LH	↑ estrogen, androgen production
FSH	↑ oocyte and sperm maturation (see Chap. 8)
GH	↑ general growth
	↓ glucose uptake into cells → diabetogenic
	↑ protein synthesis
	↑ lipolysis
	↑ IGF production in liver
PRL	↑ milk production
	↑ breast development
	Inhibition of ovulation and spermatogenesis via ↓ GnRH
ACTH	↑ glucocorticoid production (see adrenal section)

What hormone is downstream to GH that is imperative in growth and development?

Insulin-like growth factor (IGF)

Name the actions of GH that are mediated through IGF.

↑ protein synthesis in bone, muscle, and organs → ↑ linear growth, ↑ lean body mass, and ↑ organ size

When during a lifetime is GH release greatest?

During the "growth spurt" of puberty

During a 24-hour period, when is GH the highest?

Around midnight

What factors ↓ GH secretion?

1. GHRH
2. Sleep
3. Stress
4. Exercise
5. Starvation
6. Hypoglycemia

What factors ↓ GH secretion?

1. GH and IGF (negative feedback)
2. Obesity
3. Hyperglycemia
4. Somatostatins

Diagram the GH feedback loop.

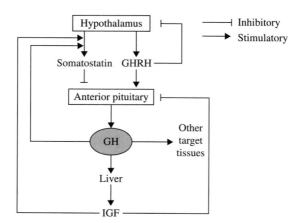

Figure 7.5   GH feedback loop.

In children, what do we call the clinical condition wherein excess GH is released?	Gigantism. The epiphyseal plates are open and children experience linear growth in excess of expected. In adults this leads to acromegaly.
What factors ↑ prolactin secretion?	Breast-feeding (most important stimulus) Stress TRH Dopamine antagonists
What factors ↓ prolactin secretion?	Dopamine (PIF)- tonic inhibition prolactin (negative feedback) Dopamine agonists (e.g., bromocriptine) SS

Diagram prolactin secretion and negative feedback.

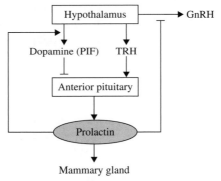

Figure 7.6   Prolactin secretion. Prolactin also inhibits GnRH which discourages the gonadal hormones and thereby pregnancy.

Name the actions of the posterior pituitary hormones.

Oxytocin	↑ contraction of myoepithelial cells in breasts (↑ milk ejection) ↑ contraction of uterus
ADH	↑ H_2O permeability of the distal tubule and collecting duct Constricts vascular smooth muscle
What type of hormones are oxytocin and ADH?	Polypeptide hormones

Where is ADH synthesized?

Supraoptic nuclei of the hypothalamus

Where are oxytocin and ADH stored and released?

Posterior pituitary

How are oxytocin and ADH synthesized and secreted?

Precursor protein
↓
Cleaved and packaged into secretory granules with neurophysins (carrier proteins)
↓
Transported by axoplasmic flow to posterior pituitary

What is the ADH receptor used in the kidney and in vascular tissue? What is its second messenger system?

Renal effect: V_2 receptor → cAMP

Smooth muscle effect: V_1 receptor → IP_3

What factors ↑ ADH secretion? (See also Chap. 5)

High serum osmolarity (directly)

Volume depletion (indirectly)

Pain (minor)

Nausea (minor)

Hypoglycemia (minor)

Nicotine (minor)

Opiates (minor)

What factors ↓ ADH secretion? (See also Chap. 5)

Low serum osmolarity
Atrial natriuretic peptide (ANP)

α-Agonists

Ethanol

How does the hypothalamus sense osmolarity changes of serum?

Specialized vessels in the region lack the standard blood-brain barrier, perivascular cells swell or shrink according to the tonicity of serum. This provides information via specialized mechanoreceptors

Where is oxytocin synthesized?

Paraventricular nuclei of the hypothalamus

What factors regulate oxytocin secretion?

Breast-feeding

Sight or sound of infant

Dilation of cervix

What effect does lithium have on the body's response to ADH?

Decreases the response through nephrogenic resistance

ADRENAL GLAND

What are the three zones of the adrenal cortex (from outer to inner zones) and what do they produce?

Zona **G**lomerulosa—Mineralocorticoids

Zona **F**asciculata—Glucocorticoids

Zona **R**eticularis—Androgens

*Remember: "**GFR**" makes "salt, sugar, sex"

What are the special cells of the adrenal medulla called?

Chromaffin cells

What are the embryological origins of chromaffin cells?

Neural crest cells

What is the product of the adrenal medulla?

Catecholamines: epinephrine (Epi), norepinephrine (NE)

What controls the release of catecholamines from the medulla?

Discussed at length in Chap. 2, but recall that the chromaffin cells, derived from neural crest cells, are simply modified postganglionic sympathetic neurons, so release of catecholamines is a consequence of CNS sympathetic discharge.

From what are the adrenocortical (steroid) hormones derived?

Cholesterol

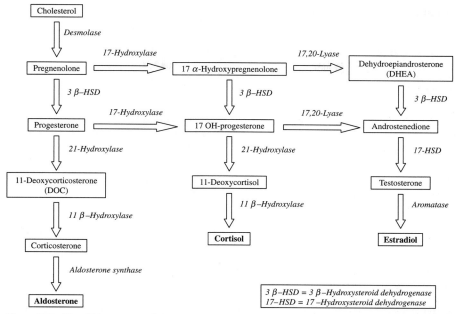

Figure 7.7 Steroid hormone pathway.

*Remember, individual layers of cortex have the portion of the pathway necessary to produce their primary hormone.

Which zone of the adrenal gland is the only producer of aldosterone synthase?	The zona glomerulosa, that is why it is the only zone to produce aldosterone
What happens when there is an enzyme deficiency in the pathway?	Steroid intermediates will accumulate above the level of the missing enzyme, and will be shunted down an alternative pathway.
What is the most common enzyme deficiency?	21 β–Hydroxylase
What steroids will be produced in excess if there is a deficiency in:	
21 β-Hydroxylase	Mineralocorticoid and glucocorticoid production is halted, and adrenal androgen production will be increased.
17 α-Hydroxylase	Decreased glucocorticoid and androgen production, increased mineralocorticoid production

What is special about the enzymes of the steroid hormone pathway?

Most are members of the cytochrome P 450 system

What is the rate-limiting step in the synthetic pathway?

Cholesterol desmolase; the initial step in all steroid pathways.

How is this step regulated?

ACTH

Name the actions of ACTH.

1. ↑ activation of desmolase
2. preferential expression of enzymes leading to cortisol synthesis
3. ↑ cholesterol uptake into adrenal cortex
4. ↑ proliferation of zona fasciculata if ACTH elevation is prolonged

What factors ↑ ACTH secretion?

1. CRH
2. Circadian rhythm-peak in the early morning
3. Emotions/stress
4. Central nervous system (CNS) trauma

What factors ↓ ACTH secretion?

Cortisol (negative feedback)

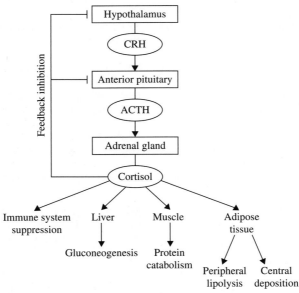

Figure 7.8   CRH, ACTH, cortisol loop.

Clinically, what is the most important stimulus for cortisol secretion?

Stress and illness; through all of the mechanisms discussed below it is the predominate counter-regulatory hormone for acute inflammation.

Name the actions of cortisol.

↑ hepatic gluconeogenesis

↓ protein synthesis

↑ protein degradation

↓ bone formation

↓ insulin sensitivity

↓ immune/inflammatory response

↓ ACTH secretion (negative feedback)

Facilitate vasoconstrictive properties of arterioles to catecholamines via alpha-1 receptor up-regulation

How does cortisol suppress the immune/ inflammatory response?

Induces the synthesis of lipocortin, which inhibits the formation of arachidonic acid

Inhibits IL-2 production

Inhibits the release of histamine and serotonin from mast cells and platelets

Name the primary actions of aldosterone.

↑ Na^+ resorption in renal distal tubules and ↑ K^+ and H^+ excretion

What factors regulate aldosterone synthesis?

1. Renin-angiotensin II-aldosterone system
2. ↑ K^+
3. Some tonic control by ACTH

Describe the renin-angiotensin-aldosterone pathway.

Decreased perfusion of the juxtaglomerular apparatus (JGA) in the kidney stimulates the release of renin. Renin cleaves the inactive peptide angiotensinogen to angiotensin I. The angiotensin converting enzyme (ACE) converts angiotensin I to the active peptide, angiotensin II, which acts as a potent vasoconstrictor and stimulates the release of aldosterone from the adrenal cortex. Aldosterone, in turn, stimulates the reabsorption of Na^+ and water, increasing blood volume.

When is the renin-angiotensin II-aldosterone system activated?

1. ↓ blood volume
2. ↓ serum Na^+

What cells monitor hyponatremia and hypovolemia to regulate renin release?

Hypovolemia is detected by arterial baroreceptors which communicate with the JGA via the nervous system. The macula densa of the distal tubule monitors sodium concentrations and communicates with the juxtaglomerular cells to release renin when that value falls.

Where is ACE found?

Lungs (major) and vasculature (minor)

What other systems are influenced by aldosterone?

Many, aldosterone works nearly everywhere sodium can be lost, so in addition to the vascular and renal systems, the GI tract and even sweat glands are affected.

How are all the above steroid hormones inactivated and excreted?

1. Catabolized by liver (majority)
2. Excreted through urine and bile/stool

From what precursor are the catecholamines derived?

Tyrosine

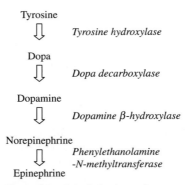

Figure 7.9 Catecholamine pathway.

How are the effects of Epi and NE mediated, and what are their second messenger systems?

Via α-and β-adrenergic receptors:

α_1 receptor $\rightarrow$ intracellular Ca^{2+}

α_2 receptor $\rightarrow$ $\downarrow$ cAMP

β_1 receptor $\rightarrow$ $\downarrow$ cAMP

β_2 receptor $\rightarrow$ $\downarrow$ cAMP

What factors regulate Epi and NE release?

(For a list of the actions of Epi and NE, please refer to Chap. 2, page 25.)
1. Sympathetic stimulation
2. Stress
3. Trauma
4. Surgery
5. Exercise
6. Hypoglycemia
7. Nicotine

What are the half-lives of Epi and NE?

Approximately 2 minutes in circulation

How are catecholamines metabolized?

Nerve endings:

$$Norepinephrine$$
$$\downarrow MAO$$
Deaminated derivatives

MAO = monoamine oxidase

Liver:

$$NE, Epi, deaminated\ derivatives$$
$$\downarrow COMT$$
$$Metanephrines \rightarrow urine$$
$$\downarrow$$
Vanillylmandelic acid (VMA) $\rightarrow$ urine

COMT = catechol-O-methyltransferase

What are the percentages of catecholamine derivatives found in urine?

~50% metanephrines

~35% VMA

The rest are other deaminated products

What is the significance of elevated VMA in the urine?

It indicates excess NE, Epi secretion. Used clinically to identify tumors of the adrenal medulla (pheochromocytoma)

THE ENDOCRINE PANCREAS

What are the pancreatic endocrine hormones?

Insulin, glucagon, and somatostatin (SS)

What metabolic process do they influence?

Serum glucose (blood glucose) regulation

How are the endocrine cells of the pancreas arranged?

The alpha, beta, and delta cells are arranged into islets of Langerhans. These have unique internal portal blood flow that allows for paracrine signaling. Also, beta cells are also linked via gap junctions to allow for rapid synchronization of insulin release.

Which cells synthesize insulin?

β-cells found in the islets of Langerhans

What type of hormone is insulin?

A polypeptide hormone

What are the steps of insulin synthesis?

Preproinsulin
↓
Proinsulin (C-peptide joins chains A and B)
↓
Insulin + C-peptide

What is the importance of C-peptide?

It distinguishes an endogenous source of insulin from an exogenous source. Used clinically when we suspect surreptitious administration of insulin (Think: the nurse with Munchausen's).

Where is insulin secreted?

Into portal circulation

How are the effects of insulin mediated?

Through insulin receptors on various tissues

What is its second messenger system?

Insulin receptor is a tyrosine kinase, which phosphorylates itself and other proteins

Name the actions of insulin in:

Skeletal and cardiac muscle

↑ glucose uptake via Glut-4 (*insulin-sensitive* glucose transporter)

↑ active transport of amino acids

↑ protein synthesis

↓ protein degradation

↑ K^+ into cells

Liver

↓ gluconeogenesis

↓ glycogenolysis

↑ glycogenesis

Adipocytes

↑ triglyceride synthesis

↓ lipolysis

What is the overall effect of insulin on serum levels of:

Glucose	Decrease
Amino acids	Decrease
Fatty acids	Decrease
Ketoacids	Decrease
K^+	Decrease

What factors regulate insulin secretion?

1. ↑ blood glucose (*primary*)
2. ↑ amino acids (especially leucine, arginine)
3. ↑ fatty acids
4. Gastric inhibitory peptide (GIP)
5. Vagus nerve stimulation
6. GH
7. SS (inhibitory effect)

How do the pancreatic β-cells *sense* serum glucose?

Via Glut-2 (*glucose sensor* glucose transporter, which is insulin *independent*)

Glucose moves through the facilitated transported, Glut-2, on β-cells
↓
Glucose metabolized to ATP
↓
β-cell membrane depolarization via ATP sensitive K^+ channel closure
↓
Insulin release from pancreas

Describe the bimodal secretion of insulin secretion in response to blood glucose?

Biphasic response:
1. Rapid burst of preformed insulin upon glucose exposure
2. Slowly rising release of freshly synthesized insulin

Describe insulin receptor regulation in:

Starvation state	Up-regulation
Obesity	Down-regulation (insulin resistance)

Where is glucagon synthesized?

α-Cells of islets of Langerhans

What type of hormone is glucagon?

A single-chain polypeptide hormone

Where in circulation is glucagon secreted?	Into portal circulation
How are the effects of glucagon mediated?	Glucagon receptor
What is its second messenger system?	cAMP

Name the actions of glucagon on:

Liver	↑ glycogenolysis ↑ gluconeogenesis ↑ lipolysis ↓ protein degradation ↓ protein synthesis
Adipocytes	↑ lipolysis

What is the overall effect of glucagon on serum levels of:

Glucose	Increase
Fatty acids	Increase
Ketoacids	Increase

What factors regulate glucagon secretion?	1. ↓ blood glucose 2. ↑ amino acids (especially arginine and leucine) 3. Epi 4. NE 5. Glucocorticoids 6. Cholecystokinin 7. SS (inhibitory)
Where is SS synthesized?	1. Delta cells of islets of Langerhans 2. Intestines 3. Nervous system
What is SS?	A polypeptide hormone—secreted in two forms
Name the actions of SS (pancreatic form).	↓ insulin ↓ glucagon ↓ gastrin
In the absence of insulin, how does the body respond?	Insulin allows the body to maintain anabolic metabolism (it can use exogenous sugar for energy). In its absence the body shifts to catabolism, mobilizing stored forms of energy. It does this acutely through the combined action of glucagon, and catecholamines.

Blood glucose regulation is primarily a balance, then, of what hormones?

Insulin versus glucagon and catecholamines

What does catabolism mean?

That the body is actively breaking down stored energy forms to use them

What stored forms of energy are broken down?

Fatty acids and proteins

What are these processes called?

Lipolysis and proteolysis

What by-products form as a result?

Ketoacids

What is the condition called that is defined by underproduction or absence of insulin?

Type 1 diabetes

What are the prototypic symptoms of diabetes?

Polydipsia, polyuria, and weight loss

Describe the physiology behind that constellation of symptoms:

When a type 1 diabetes takes in a large glucose load, that makes its way to the bloodstream. Without insulin to facilitate its entry into cells, it builds up in the blood stream. As glucagon begins to be released, the insulin-glucagon scale tips towards glucagon and cellular machinery switches to catabolism, generating cellular by-products of lipolysis and proteolysis leading to depletion of cellular stores and weight loss.

The glucose in the blood acts as an osmotic force drawing water from the intracellular space, which is freely filtered at the glomerulus and incompletely reabsorbed, it pulls water through the renal tubule and leads to polydipsia.

THYROID GLAND

What chemical element is required for normal thyroid function?

Iodine

What is it used for?

Thyroid hormone (TH) is heavily iodinated, without iodine the body is incapable of producing functional TH.

Where are thyroid hormones synthesized?	Follicular cells of the thyroid gland
What protein is the precursor to thyroid hormone?	Thyroglobulin—contains the iodotyrosyl residues monoiodotyrosine (MIT) and diiodotyrosine (DIT)
What is meant by "colloid"?	Follicular cells form a sphere, the inside of this sphere contains iodine, and thyroglobulin, along with the enzyme thyroid peroxidase.
Name the two active thyroid hormones.	1. T_4 (thyroxine)—most abundant 2. T_3 (3,5,3'-triiodothyronine)—most active
What are the steps of thyroid hormone synthesis?	1. Inorganic iodide (I^-) actively transported into follicular cell → diffuse into colloid/lumen → oxidized to iodine (I_2) via thyroid peroxidase 2. Thyroglobulin produced in rough ER of follicular cell → secreted into colloid 3. In colloid, I_2 is incorporated into tyrosine residues of thyroglobulin → MIT and DIT formed Coupling of MIT and DIT residue occurs, forming T_3 (MIT + DIT), reverse T_3, or T_4 (DIT + DIT). These are, however, still linked to thyroglobulin.

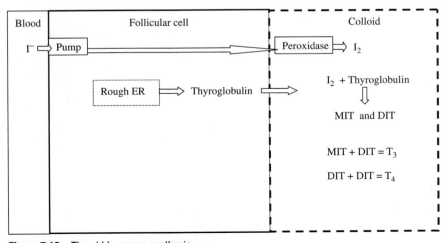

Figure 7.10   Thyroid hormone synthesis.

What are the steps of thyroid hormone secretion?	1. Thyroglobulin is taken into follicular cell → colloid filled endocytic vesicles fuse with lysosomes hydrolyzed into T_3, T_4, DIT, MIT 2. T_3 and T_4 secreted into plasma 3. DIT and MIT deiodinated → tyrosines
Where else are thyroid hormones produced?	Nowhere, but 80% of T_3 is made through peripheral conversion of T4 in tissues, especially liver and kidney
What else does T_4 form peripherally?	T_4 → deiodinated → inactive reverse T_3 (rT_3)
Why is rT_3 inactive?	Inappropriate removal of iodine leaves a molecule that is sterically incapable of binding to the thyroid hormone receptor
How do thyroid hormones circulate?	>99% of hormone in circulation is bound to protein (e.g., thyroxine-binding globulins [TBG], albumin, and prealbumin) The minority of thyroid hormone circulates freely.
What are the half-lives of T_3 and T_4?	T_3: 1 day T_4: 7 days

Name the actions of thyroid hormone on:

Metabolism	↑ basal metabolic rate (BMR), ↑ O_2 consumption, ↑ heat production, activate Na^+-K^+-ATPase ↑ glucose absorption, glycogenolysis, gluconeogenesis, glucose oxidation ↑ lipolysis and protein degradation
Growth/development	Required for actions of GH to promote linear growth/bone formation Stimulate bone maturation Required for fetal CNS development-involved in myelin and synapse formation
Cardiac	↑ β-adrenergic receptors → ↑ cardiac output (HR × SV) ↑ systolic blood pressure only
Respiratory	↑ ventilation rate
Reproductive	Required for ovary and testis maturation

What factors regulate thyroid hormone synthesis and secretion?	Thyrotropin releasing hormone (TRH) and TSH
What is TSH?	A glycoprotein with α- and β-subunit
Where is TSH synthesized?	Anterior pituitary
How are the effects of TSH mediated?	Through TSH receptor on follicular cells
What is its second messenger system?	cAMP
What are the actions of TSH?	Increase all aspects of thyroid hormone synthesis and secretion as well as exerting a trophic effect on the thyroid tissue
Where is TRH synthesized?	Paraventricular nuclei of the hypothalamus
What is its second messenger system?	IP_3
What are the actions of TRH?	↑ pituitary secretion of TSH

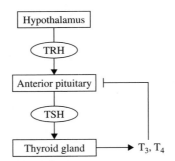

T_3, T_4 offers feedback to the anterior pituitary which leads to down regulation of the TRH receptor

Figure 7.11   TRH, TSH, and thyroid hormone loop.

PARATHYROID GLAND

Name some of the physiological processes that involve Ca^{2+}.	Muscular contraction
	Membrane permeability
	Endocrine and exocrine secretions
	Enzyme regulation
	Coagulation

How does Ca^{2+} circulate in serum?

50% to 60% in free, ionized form (biologically active)

40% bound to plasma proteins or complexed to other ions

Where is Ca^{2+} stored and approximately in what amounts?

ECF: 0.9 g (less that 0.1%)

ICF: 11 g (about 1%)

Bone: 1000 g (the rest)

How is Ca^{2+} stored in bones?

Two-thirds as inorganic crystals = hydroxyapatite (Ca$_{10}$[PO$_4$]$_6$[OH]$_2$)

One-third as organic materials (e.g., Ca$_2$PO$_4$)

Name the three organs that play an important role in serum Ca^{2+} regulation.

1. Intestines → absorption
2. Kidney → excretion
3. Bone → long-term storage

How is Ca^{2+} homeostasis maintained?

Net absorption must be balanced by excretion

Diagram Ca^{2+} metabolism including its relationship to the gut, the kidney, and bone.

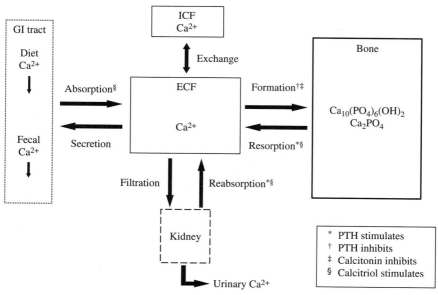

Figure 7.12 Ca^{2+} metabolism.

Name the three primary hormones that play an important role in Ca^{2+} homeostasis.	1. Parathyroid hormone (PTH) 2. Calcitriol (1,25-dihydroxyvitamin D) 3. Calcitonin
What type of hormone is PTH?	A polypeptide hormone
Where is PTH synthesized and secreted?	Chief cells of the four parathyroid glands
What factors regulates PTH secretion?	Serum Ca^{2+} (negative feedback), Mg^{2+}
What happens to PTH secretion when:	
Serum Ca^{2+} is low	Increase
Serum Ca^{2+} is high	Decrease
How do magnesium levels influence PTH secretion?	Suppresses PTH and encourages calcium deposition in storage.
How are the effects of PTH mediated?	Directly on bone and kidney through the PTH receptors, and indirectly in the intestines via indirect activation of vitamin D
What is its second messenger system?	cAMP and intracellular Ca^{2+}
Name the actions of PTH on the following:	
Kidney	↑ Ca^{2+} reabsorption →↑ serum Ca^{2+} (distal tubule) ↓ PO^{4-} reabsorption → limits calcium sequestration in bone → ↑ serum Ca^{2+} (in the proximal tubule) ↑ 1 α-hydroxylase →↑ calcitriol production → ↑ serum Ca^{2+} (proximal tubule)
Bone	Stimulates osteoclasts to increase bone resorption → ↑ Ca$_2$PO$_4$ in ECF Inhibits osteoblasts (directly and indirectly) to further increase bone resorption
What is vitamin D (cholecalciferol)?	A steroid hormone that utilizes a UV radiation mediated reaction for final activation
What is the active form of vitamin D?	Calcitriol (1,25-dihydroxycholecalciferol)
What are the inactive forms of vitamin D?	1. Cholecalciferol 2. 25-Hydroxycholecalciferol 3. 24,25-Hydroxycholecalciferol

Where and how is calcitriol synthesized?

Vitamin D

$\downarrow$ 25-Hydroxylase (liver)

25-Hydroxycholecalciferol

$\downarrow$ 1 α-Hydroxylase (kidney)

1,25-Hydroxycholecalciferol

What factors regulate calcitriol synthesis?

Activity of 1 α-hydroxylase, which is $\uparrow$ by

$\downarrow$ serum Ca^{2+}

$\uparrow$ PTH levels

$\downarrow$ serum PO^{4-}

Note that the final activation of vitamin D is poorly regulated because it is dependent on sun exposure

How are the effects of calcitriol mediated? Through the calcitriol receptor

What type of hormone is calcitonin? A polypeptide hormone

Name the actions of calcitriol on:

    Intestines

Induces Ca^{2+}-binding protein $\rightarrow$ $\uparrow$ absorption Ca^{2+}

$\uparrow$ PO^{4+} reabsorption

    Kidney $\uparrow$ Ca^{2+} and PO^{4-} reabsorption

    Bone $\uparrow$ bone resorption $\rightarrow \uparrow$ serum Ca_2 and PO^{4-}

Where is calcitonin synthesized and secreted?

Parafollicular cells (C cells) of thyroid gland

What factor regulates calcitonin secretion?

$\uparrow$ serum Ca^{2+} stimulates its secretion

What is its second messenger system? cAMP

What is the action of calcitonin? $\downarrow$ bone resorption by osteoclasts

Summarize the events that regulate the following hormone secretions:

    PTH $\downarrow$ serum Ca^{2+}

    Calcitriol

$\downarrow$ serum Ca^{2+}

$\uparrow$ PTH levels

$\downarrow$ serum PO^{4-}

    Calcitonin $\uparrow$ serum Ca^{2+}

Summarize the actions of the Ca^{2+} homeostasis hormones at each site:

Intestines

PTH: ↑ Ca^{2+} absorption through activating calcitriol (minor)

Calcitriol: ↑ Ca^{2+} and PO^{4-} reabsorption (major)

Calcitonin: no effect

Kidney

PTH: ↑ Ca^{2+} reabsorption and ↓ PO^{4-} reabsorption (major)

Calcitriol: ↑ Ca^{2+} and PO^{4+} reabsorption (minor)

Calcitonin: no effect

Bone

PTH: ↑ resorption (major)

Calcitriol: ↑ resorption (minor)

Calcitonin: ↓ resorption

CLINICAL VIGNETTES

An elderly woman presents to her primary care physician (PCP) for evaluation. She is complaining of abdominal discomfort and constipation for the past 6 months. During this time, she thinks her arthritis has gotten worse, as her "bones and joints" seem to be aching throughout the day, and she thinks that this is making her feel more depressed. Her past medical history is significant for hypertension controlled with a thiazide diuretic, gastroesophageal reflux controlled with TUMS, and recurrent kidney stones. What is the likely etiology of this patient's disease?

Hypercalcemia secondary to thiazide and antacid use. Remember the signs of hypercalcemia: stones, bones, abdominal groans, and psychiatric overtones!

A 24-year-old female with an extensive psychiatric history, presents to the ED with insidious onset of headache, double vision, and nausea. Upon further questioning, she states she has not had a menstrual period for the past 4 months but has noted a milky discharge from both her nipples. A pregnancy test is negative. What should you suspect?

Prolactinoma

How does this explain the amenorrhea?

High levels of prolactin inhibit the secretion of GnRH, which in turn leads to decreased secretion of LH and FSH.

A 58-year-old man with diagnosed small-cell lung cancer, has begun to experience polyuria and polydipsia. He presents to your office due to weakness and fatigue. Laboratory results reveal he is severely hyponatremic. You suspect this patient is suffering from paraneoplastic SIADH. What further evidence would aid in your diagnosis and how would you treat it?

SIADH is a diagnosis of exclusion.
   a. Hyponatremia in the face of inappropriately concentrated urine
   b. Volume expansion without edema
   c. Plasma osmolarity below 270
   d. Low BUN and creatinine
   e. Measurement of plasma and urine ADH levels
   f. Treatment involves water restriction and the search for the underlying cause

What is the danger of correcting hyponatremia too quickly?

A rapid flux of water into the ECF can cause central pontine myelinolysis. The way to think of this is that as the relatively hyperosmolar ECF pulls water out of neurons, that moving water sometime rips and tears the myelin away from the neuron (it is actually far more complex, but it helps to remember the phenomenon).

Symptoms include para or quadriparesis, diplopia, dysphagia, and other neurologic abnormalities. Sodium replacement generally should not exceed 0.5 mEq/L per hour.

A 42-year-old female presents to your office for follow up evaluation of a compression fracture of the T10/T11 vertebrae. She states the injury resulted from a fall she sustained after feeling weak while trying to climb the stairs. As you inspect the patient, you note a mildly obese female, with fat distribution largely around the trunk and posterior neck. Purple striae are noted on the abdomen, bruises scattered throughout her extremities, and hirsutism (male pattern hair development) on the face. What is high on your differential diagnosis and how does this relate to the presenting vertebral fracture?

Cushing disease. High cortisol levels can lead to osteoporosis, impaired collagen production, and protein catabolism, offering explanation for the bruising, muscle weakness, and fracture. The most common cause is iatrogenic, with the use of high dose steroids. That is absent in this woman, so one must think of tumors leading to cortisol secretion, which can develop in any part of the pituitary-adrenal axis. Confirmation is done with laboratory testing that will reveal high levels of both ACTH and cortisol if primary (coming from the pituitary adenoma), or just high cortisol with suppressed ACTH (if from an adrenal source).

This woman's fracture is clearly a consequence of her osteoporotic bones.

A 34-year-old male presents to the ED with a sudden, severe headache. He states he was working his normal route as a mail carrier, when all of the sudden he became sweaty and felt his heart palpitating. He soon developed a severe headache, and collapsed to the ground. A bystander witnessed the events and called an ambulance. He reports this has happened a few times, but never this severe. Vital signs reveal a blood pressure of 205/130 and a heart rate of 118. What could be causing this clinical picture?

Pheochromocytoma. Remember the 5 P's: Pressure, Pain, Palpitations, Pallor, and Perspiration.

A 35-year-old female presents to PCP with a 1-week history of palpitations and diarrhea. She reports that over the past 2 months, she has experienced a 15 lbs weight loss, despite normal appetite and food intake. She also describes having difficulty sleeping. Physical examination reveals exophthalmos, warm-moist skin, and a diffusely enlarged, symmetric, and non-tender thyroid. Laboratory results revealed a low TSH and elevated free T_3/T_4. What is the likely diagnosis?

Graves disease. In this disease the thyroid receives autoimmune stimulation leading to excessive release of thyroid hormones.

A 40-year-old female presents to your office with a 2-month history of fatigue. She has experienced a 20-lb weight gain over the past 3 to 4 months. She thinks this could partly be due to her depressed mood and lack of energy to exercise. Patient reports no other symptoms aside from occasional constipation. The physical examination is unremarkable. A thyroid function panel reveals an elevated TSH. What is the likely diagnosis and how would you confirm?

Hashimoto thyroiditis; confirm with antithyroglobulin antibodies or antimicrosomal antibodies

Probing would likely reveal that prior to her recent hypothyroid symptoms, she had previously had symptoms of hyperthyroidism. During early disease the overstimulated thyroid releases its hormonal payload. Late in disease the gland "burns out" and slowly fails to function.

A 32-year-old male with a 15-year history of extensive alcohol use presents with foul-smelling stool and epigastric pain that radiates to the back and relieved by sitting upright or leaning forward. Physical examination shows pallor. This is his 10th presentation with this type of presentation. His workup reveals normal lipase and elevated glucose. Why does he have elevated glucose?

Glucose intolerance occurs frequently in chronic pancreatitis, which is likely due to a decrease in pancreatic insulin reserve or in insulin responsiveness

A man recently presented to his primary care provider with a complaint of impotence. Upon examination, the patient is found to also have galactorrhea. He is sent for an MRI, which confirms the diagnosis of a prolactinoma. What medication is used to treat him and why?

Bromocriptine, it is a dopamine agonist. This enhances the action of dopamine on the anterior pituitary. Remember that dopamine, in this endocrine loop, is also called prolactin inhibiting factor. In these patients, bromocriptine is used as first line therapy and often the prolactinoma undergoes hypoplasia with loss of total volume.

An elderly male has come to his PCP with a complaint of straining to urinate. After a thorough interview and examination, it is found that the patient suffers from benign prostatic hypertrophy. What kind of medications will the doctor most likely prescribe and why?

5 α-reductase inhibitors, they block the activation of testosterone to dihydrotestosterone in the prostate, which helps to reduce prostate volume.

Incidentally, they may also help him with male pattern baldness, also though to be a product of testosterone interaction with hair follicles.

The next three questions refer to the following vignette: A patient comes into the ER with complaints of sweating, heart palpitations, and recent weight loss. Tests show that the patient is suffering from hyperthyroidism. Surgery is not an option. What medication would be used for treatment and why?

Propylthiouracil, it inhibits the peroxidase enzyme

If the above patient is found to have Graves disease, what is the underlying physiology?

The body has begun to generate antibodies that stimulate the TSH receptor in the thyroid gland oversecretes hormone.

In the above case, what would be the values seen on thyroid function tests (TFTs)?

$\downarrow$ thyroid stimulating hormone (TSH), $\uparrow T_3$, and $\uparrow T_4$

A patient comes into his PCP complaining that she is gaining weight on her face. Her examination reveals a hypertensive female with a round face, and striae on her abdomen. Her laboratory reports are significant for hyperglycemia, high cortisol, and androgen levels. What hormone can be measured to differentiate Cushing syndrome, any disease leading to primary hyperaldosteronism, from Cushing disease, also called secondary hyperaldosteronism?

Adrenocorticotropic hormone (ACTH), it is high in Cushing disease and low in Cushing syndrome. Cushing syndrome results from either administration of pharmacologic doses of glucocorticoids, or less likely, bilateral hyperplasia of the adrenal glands

A patient is found to be hypertensive, hypokalemic, in metabolic alkalosis, and has decreased renin secretion. What disease is this patient suffering from?

Conn syndrome (e.g., hyperaldosteronism) High aldosterone leads to:

Increased Na^+ reabsorption, which increases the ECF $\rightarrow$ hypertension

Increased K^+ secretion

Increased H^+ secretion

Increased ECF and blood pressure (BP) leads to inhibition of renin secretion

An 8-year-old boy is brought to the doctor by his parents who are concerned about the recent changes that he has undergone. It is found that he has all the signs of early puberty. What enzyme is most likely responsible for these changes?

21 β-Hydroxylase deficiency. Without this enzyme there is an excess secretion of aldosterone and sex hormones, but no production of cortisol and estradiol. Refer to Fig. 7.7 (page 211).

A 17-year-old woman presents to the ER with syncope. While doing the initial assessment, it is found that the patient is hypertensive and has no axillary hair. The cause of the syncope is found to be secondary to her hypoglycemia. Additional laboratory reports on the patient show that she is hypokalemic, and has a metabolic alkalosis. What enzyme deficiency is responsible for the above findings?

17 α-Hydroxylase deficiency. The lack of axillary hair (and pubic hair) is a result from a lack of adrenal androgens. The hypoglycemia is from the decreased glucocorticoids. The metabolic alkalosis, hypokalemia, and hypertension are a result of the increased aldosterone.

While studying the pancreas, a researcher injects CCK into a patient. What hormone from the pancreas will be found at a higher level after the injection?

Glucagon

A 16-year-old girl is found by her parents in her bedroom passed out. They call 911. Emergency medical technicians arrive on the scene and find the girl to have a glucose level of 25. They begin an infusion of glucose and bring her to the hospital. By the time they reach the hospital, the patient wakes up. She refuses to speak and does not want to talk about the episode. Initial tests find the girl to have very high insulin levels, but very low protein C levels. What is the most likely etiology of the patient's hypoglycemia?

Exogenous injection of insulin. Protein C is a marker for insulin production. If this were a result from an insulinoma, the level of protein C would also be very high.

Surreptitious administration of insulin should direct us toward psychiatric evaluation.

A young man is brought to the ER poorly responsive. He is found to be hypotensive and tachypneic. His breath has a fruity smell. Laboratory reports show severe hyperglycemia, hyperkalemia, and metabolic acidosis. What is wrong with this patient? Explain the patient's symptoms.

The patient has classic case of diabetic ketoacidosis from uncontrolled diabetes mellitus.

Hyperglycemia—insulin deficiency

Hypotension—ECF volume contraction resulting from high-filtered load of glucose exceeds the kidney's reabsorptive capacity

Metabolic acidosis—secondary from the excess production of ketoacids

Hyperkalemia—lack of insulin (insulin promotes K^+ reabsorption)

A 6-year-old boy is brought to his pediatrician by his worried parents because he is shorter than all his school mates. The boy's parents are of average height. What blood tests can the pediatrician order to rule out an endocrine cause of his short stature?

GH and insulin-like growth factor (IGF), as well as TSH and T_4. Both GH deficiency and hypothyroidism can result in deficits in linear growth.

A pregnant woman with hypothyroidism asks her obstetrician if levothyroxine (synthetic T_4) is safe to take during pregnancy. What is her doctor's response?

It is safe and essential to continue synthetic T_4 therapy during pregnancy for all women with hypothyroidism. Thyroid hormones are important for fetal central nervous system (CNS) development.

What happens to steroid hormone levels in patients with liver disease?

The liver metabolizes the majority of steroid hormones in the body. In liver disease, steroid levels increase because the rate of hepatic inactivation is diminished.

An 8-year-old boy is brought to the doctor by his concerned parents, because he has recently undergone many changes resembling the signs of puberty. Describe the possible problems along the hypothalamic-pituitary-adrenal/gonadal axis that could be responsible for these changes?

Hypothalamus: excess GnRH

Pituitary: excess FSH and LH

Testes: excess testosterone

Adrenal glands: excess steroid hormones

Excess hormones, in general, are due to a hormone-secreting tumor in the associated organ.

For the boy in the previous vignette, what adrenal enzyme problems may lead to similar symptoms?

21-Hydroxylase deficiency or 11 β-hydroxylase deficiency, which are the two most common causes of congenital adrenal hyperplasia (CAH). CAH is characterized by deficient cortisol and/or aldosterone and excess sex hormones. These enzyme deficiencies result in excessive steroid hormone precursors, which then enter the androgen pathway and lead to excess sex hormones.

A woman in her third trimester of pregnancy is worried that her baby has not moved in the past 36 hours or so. What hormone can be measured to determine fetal well-being?

Serum or urinary estriol. Estriol is made by the placenta from dehydroepiandrosterone-S (DHEA-S), which is made by fetal adrenal glands.

An elderly widow complains of muscle twitches and numbness and tingling around her mouth. On further questioning, the patient admits she has not been eating very well since her husband's death 10 months ago, and she does not go outside very much. What laboratory tests can reveal the etiology of her numbness and tingling?

Serum Ca^{2+} and vitamin D levels may help establish a diagnosis of hypocalcemia. Her hypocalcemia most likely results from poor nutritional intake of calcium and is worsened by vitamin D deficiency from lack of exposure to UV light (vitamin D is important for calcium absorption from the intestines).

Hypocalcemia symptoms include muscle cramps or tetany, perioral paresthesias, seizure, and osteoporosis.

A 71-year-old woman with hypertension comes to her PCP for an annual checkup. She notes that she has recently been experiencing abdominal discomfort, constipation, heartburn, and joint pain. She takes hydrochlorothiazide and TUMS. How might her symptoms be explained?

Hypercalcemia secondary to thiazide and antacid (calcium carbonate) use. Hypercalcemia symptoms include calcium oxalate kidney stones, osteoporosis or pseudogout, constipation, peptic ulcer disease, depression, or altered consciousness.

*Remember: stones, bones, groans, abdominal moans, and psychiatric overtones

For the above patient, what is her expected parathyroid hormone (PTH), calcitriol, and calcitonin levels?

PTH: decreased

Calcitriol: decreased

Calcitonin: increased

A 3-year-old female known with a deletion of phenylalanine at position Δ F508 presents with a 2-week history of foul-smelling, large fatty stools, and difficulty gaining weight. What is the underling cause of her malabsorption?

Ninety percent of patients with cystic fibrosis have pancreatic insufficiency. The insufficiency results from thickened mucus in the pancreatic ducts, causing obstruction and ultimately autodigestion of the pancreas by activated enzymes.

Table 7.1 Overview of Hormones

Hormone	Abbreviation	Origin	Secondary Messenger	Action
Thyrotropin-releasing hormone	TRH	Hypothalamus	IP_3	Stimulates secretion of TSH and prolactin
Corticotropin-releasing hormone	CRH	Hypothalamus	cAMP	Stimulates secretion of ACTH
Gonadotropin releasing hormone	GnRH	Hypothalamus	IP_3	Stimulates LH and FSH secretion
Growth hormone releasing hormone	GHRH	Hypothalamus	IP_3	Stimulates secretion of GH
Somatostatin	SS	Hypothalamus		Inhibits secretion of GH
Prolactin inhibiting factor (dopamine)	PIF	Hypothalamus		Inhibits secretion of prolactin
Thyroid stimulating hormone	TSH	Anterior pituitary	cAMP	Stimulate synthesis and secretion of thyroid hormones
Follicle stimulating hormone	FSH	Anterior pituitary	cAMP	Stimulates oocyte and sperm maturation
Lutenizing hormone	LH	Anterior pituitary	cAMP	Stimulates ovulation, corpus luteum formation, and production of estrogen, progesterone, and androgens

(*Continued*)

Table 7.1 Overview of Hormones (Continued)

Hormone	Abbreviation	Origin	Secondary Messenger	Action
Growth hormone	GH	Anterior pituitary		Stimulates protein synthesis and growth
Prolactin	PRL	Anterior pituitary		Stimulates milk production and breast development
Adrenocorticotropic hormone	ACTH	Anterior pituitary		Stimulates synthesis and secretion of adrenal cortical hormones
Melanocyte stimulating hormone	MSH	Anterior pituitary	cAMP	Stimulates melanin synthesis
Oxytocin		Posterior pituitary	IP_3	Milk ejection and uterus contraction
Antidiuretic hormone	ADH	Posterior pituitary	V_1 receptor- IP_3 V_2 receptor- cAMP	Stimulates water reabsorption in renal collecting ducts
Thyroxine, Triiodothyronine	T4,T3	Thyroid gland		Skeletal growth; ↑ O_2 consumption; heat production; ↑ protein, fat, and carbohydrate use; perinatal maturation of CNS
Glucocorticoid (cortisol)		Adrenal cortex	steroid	Stimulates gluconeogenesis; anti-inflammatory; immunosuppressive
Estradiol		Ovary	steroid	Development of female reproductive organs; follicular phase of menstrual cycle

Hormone		Mechanism	Actions
Progesterone		steroid	Luteal phase of menstrual cycle
Testosterone		steroid	Spermatogenesis; secondary male sex characteristics
Parathyroid hormone	PTH	cAMP	↑ serum Ca^{2+}; ↓ serum phosphate
Calcitonin		cAMP	↓ serum Ca^{2+}
Aldosterone		steroid	↑ renal Na reabsorption; ↑ renal K secretion; ↑ renal H secretion
1,25 dihydroxycholecalciferol		steroid	↑ intestinal Ca absorption; ↑ bone mineralization
Insulin		tyrosine kinase	↓ blood glucose, aa, and fatty acid concentrations
Glucagon		cAMP	↑ blood glucose and fatty acid concentrations

(Gland column: Progesterone — Ovary; Testosterone — Testes; Parathyroid hormone — Parathyroid gland; Calcitonin — Thyroid gland C cells; Aldosterone — Adrenal cortex; 1,25 dihydroxycholecalciferol — Kidney; Insulin — Pancreas; Glucagon — Pancreas)

CHAPTER 8

Reproductive Physiology

DEVELOPMENT

What determines sexual differentiation? The composition of the sex chromosomes, either XY or XX corresponding to male and female phenotypes, respectively

What is gonadal sex? Presence of testes in ♂ or ovaries in ♀

What is phenotypic or somatic sex? Characteristics of internal/external genitalia

On a genomic level, what is it that determines sex? The presence of the Y chromosome. It contains the SRY gene which redirects development.

What are the names of the two parallel duct systems which develop in the fetus?
1. The mesonephric (wolffian) duct system
2. The paramesonephric (müllerian) duct system

What cells give rise to the primitive gonad? Primordial germ cells migrate from the yolk sac to the genital ridge

What factor determines ♀ gonadal sex? Absence of testicular differentiation factor (TDF): embryonic *indifferent gonads* automatically become ovaries

What three factors (or absence of factors) determine ♀ phenotypic sex?
1. Absence of MIF: müllerian duct develops into uterus, fallopian tubes, and upper vagina
2. Estrogen: stimulates urogenital sinus and tubercle to differentiate into lower vagina, clitoris, and vulva
3. Absence of TDF: embryonic *indifferent gonads* automatically become ovaries

What factor determines ♂ gonadal sex?   TDF, produced by Y chromosome

What three factors determine ♂ phenotypic sex?
1. Müllerian inhibiting factor (MIF): inhibits paramesonephric (müllerian) duct from developing into uterus and fallopian tubes
2. Testosterone: stimulates mesonephric (wolffian) duct to differentiate into epididymis, seminal vesicles, and vas deferens
3. Dihydrotestosterone (DHT): stimulates urogenital sinus and tubercle to differentiate into penis, urethra, prostate, and scrotum

Describe the process of male sexual differentiation.

Presence of SRY gene
↓
Leydig and Sertoli development
↓
Testosterone and müllerian inhibiting factor (MIF)
↓
Regression of the paramesonephric duct
↓
External genitalia differentiation

When during gestation do the testes descend into the scrotum?   During the last trimester; it requires the secretion of fetal gonadotropins

What condition describes the failure of testicular descent?   Cryptorchidism

What is the final stage in sexual development called?   Puberty

What endocrine event starts puberty?   Pulsatile increase in luteinizing hormone and follicle-stimulating hormone secretion

What regulatory event allows puberty to begin?   During childhood, gonodotropin-releasing hormone (GnRH) secretion is tonically suppressed. In adolescence it is secreted in a pulsatile pattern which promotes pubertal development.

Name some of the phenotypic changes that characterize puberty (more discussed later).   Pubic hair growth (pubarche), breast enlargement (thelarche), growth spurt, development of secondary sexual characteristics, etc.

MALE REPRODUCTIVE PHYSIOLOGY

Why do the testes descend into the scrotum?

To maintain temperature ~2°C below core body temperature, which is vital for normal spermatogenesis

Name the anatomic components of the testis and their associated function(s).

Seminiferous tubules (85% testis mass): spermatogenesis by Sertoli and germ cells

Rete testis: connects tubules and efferent ductules

Efferent ductules: transports sperm to epididymis by ciliary motion and contraction

Epididymis: reservoir and site of further morphologic and functional changes to sperm

Vas deferens: propels sperm into urethra by muscular contractions

What is the blood-testes barrier?

Tight junctions that protect spermatogenesis by preventing movement of immunologic proteins from circulation to the lumen of the seminiferous tubules

Why is the blood-testes barrier so important?

The process of meiosis leads to genetic reorganization and novel protein expression and production. This barrier is important in protecting the testes from autoimmune disruption.

Which cell type in the testis is the precursor to the male gamete?

Germ cells

Describe spermatogenesis.

Three general phases:
1. Proliferation of spermatogonia
2. Generation of genetic diversity
3. Maturation of sperm

Spermatogonium (primitive germ cell)
↓
1° spermatocyte (occurs in adolescence)
↓ *meiotic division*
2° spermatocyte
↓
Spermatid
↓ *time*
Spermatozoa (mature sperm)

What hormone most influences spermatogenesis?

Testosterone

What cell in the seminiferous tubule secretes testosterone?

Leydig cell

What cells primarily anchor and support the developing spermatid?

Sertoli cells (historically they were referred to as "nurse" cells)

What important hormone is secreted by Sertoli cells and increases testosterone concentrations in the seminiferous tubules?

Androgen-binding protein (ABP); this allows local concentrations of testosterone to be dramatically higher than systemic concentrations

Which two anterior pituitary hormones are responsible for regulating the testosterone and ABP secretion described above?

1. LH
2. FSH

LH stimulates Leydig cells (Luteinizing—Leydig) to secrete testosterone; FSH stimulates Sertoli cells to secrete ABP

Describe the negative feedback that influences this endocrine cycle.

Testosterone directly feeds back to inhibit LH secretion. The Sertoli cell secretes inhibin which then exerts negative influence over the anterior pituitary.

How long does it take for spermatogonia to mature into spermatozoa?

~74 days

How is testosterone synthesized?

Cholesterol

$\downarrow$ *cholesterol desmolase*

Pregnenolone

$\downarrow$ *17 α-hydroxylase*

17-hydroxy-pregnenolone

$\downarrow$ *17, 20-lyase*

DHEA

$\downarrow$ *3 β-hydroxysteroid DH**

Androstenedione

$\downarrow\uparrow$ *21 β-hydroxylase*

Testosterone

*DH = dehydrogenase

Name the actions of testosterone.

Embryonic differentiation of wolffian ducts to ♂ reproductive tract

Puberty

♂ secondary sexual characteristics

Contribute to Sertoli cells' maintenance of spermatogenesis

What are the ♂ secondary sexual characteristics influenced by testosterone?

Growth of penis, epididymis, vas deferens, and prostate

Growth spurt

Voice changes

↑ muscle mass

↑ sex drive

What factors regulate testosterone secretion?

1. GnRH
2. LH
3. Testosterone (negative feedback)

Diagram the hypothalamus-pituitary-gonadal (HPG) axis of testosterone.

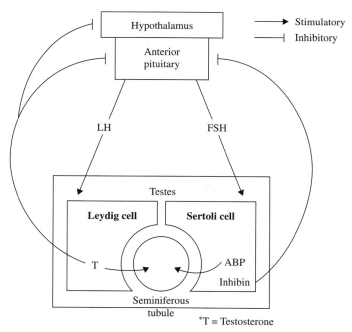

Figure 8.1 HPG axis.

Name the ♂ accessory genitalia and their associated functions.

Seminal vesicles: provides fructose to nourish sperm and secretes 60% of semen fluid volume

Prostate: secretes 20% of semen fluid volume

Bulbourethral (Cowper) and urethral (Littre) glands: lubricate sperm transit through urethra

What is the relationship between testosterone and DHT?

Testosterone

↓ *5-α-reductase*

DHT

Where is 5-α-reductase found?

Many tissues, especially the prostate

Name the actions of DHT.

Embryonic differentiation of urogenital sinus/tubercle to ♂ genitalia

♂ secondary sexual characteristics: male hair distribution

Growth of seminal vesicles

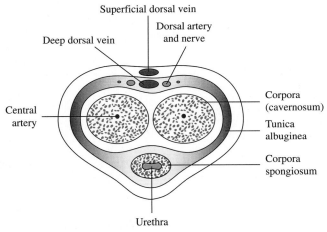

Figure 8.2 Section of the penis.

What portions of the above diagram are considered erectile tissue?

Only the corpus cavernosum.

Describe the process of erection.

With sexual stimulation, the parasympathetic system activates leading to relaxation of the vascular smooth muscle found in the penis. This relaxation leads to penile engorgement.

What anatomical feature encourages penile engorgement?	The deep fascia of the penis. These provide a fixed volume for the penis and as arterial inflow engorges the corpora, the veins in the tunica and within the corpora become compressed restricting venous outflow and increasing penile rigidity.
Is there a difference in the deep fascia as it encircles the corpora spongiosum and the corpora cavernosum?	Yes, the corpora cavernosum are ensheathed in a thicker layer of fascia which facilitates rigidity. The corporus spongiosum receives a much thinner fibrous surround allowing the urethra to maintain patency during erection. Classically, the spongiosum is *not* considered erectile tissue for this reason.
What molecular transmitter is most significant in this vascular control?	Nitric oxide (NO)
What process involves sequential contraction of the smooth muscle of the vas deferens, prostate, and seminal vesicles?	Ejaculation
Is this *particular* process mediated by the sympathetic or parasympathetic nervous systems?	The sympathetic nervous system

OVARY AND PLACENTA

Name the major anatomical components of the female reproductive tract.	Vulva and the vagina Cervix (the lowermost portion of the uterus) Uterus (body and fundus) Fallopian tubes Ovaries
Name the four cell types of the ovary and their associated product(s).	1. Theca cell: testosterone 2. Granulosa cell: estradiol (from testosterone) 3. Primordial follicle: mature ovum for ovulation 4. Luteal cell (of corpus luteum): progesterone

What enzyme converts testosterone to estradiol?

Aromatase

Describe the menstrual and oogenesis cycle:

Follicular (proliferative) phase

Days 1 to 14 (variable):
1. Estradiol ↑ and progesterone ↓
2. FSH and LH ↓ (negative feedback)
3. FSH and LH receptors ↑ (up-regulation)
4. Multiple primordial follicles enlarge (only one becomes the graafian follicle, others undergo atresia)

Ovulation

Day 15:

$$\text{Estradiol } \uparrow$$
$$\downarrow$$
$$\text{Positive feedback}$$
$$\downarrow$$
$$\text{LH surge}$$
$$\downarrow$$
$$\text{Ovulation!}$$

This phenomenon is known as the *estrogen-induced LH surge*

Temporary estradiol ↓ after ovulation

Luteal (secretory) phase

Days 15 to 28 (fixed):
1. Progesterone ↑ and estradiol ↑
2. Corpus luteum matures and produces progesterone
3. Endometrium vascularity builds to prepare for implantation of fertilized ovum
4. Corpus luteum regresses if no fertilization occurs → ↓ progesterone and ↓ estradiol

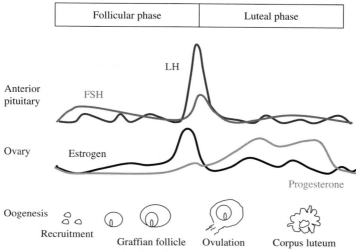

| Follicular phase | Luteal phase |

Figure 8.3   Menstrual and oogenesis cycle.

Why is the luteal phase fixed in duration?

Corpus luteum has a fixed 14-day life span

How long is the typical menstrual cycle?

Average of 28 days

When does menstruation occur?

Onset of menses marks Day 1 of menstrual cycle

What is menstruation?

Sloughing of endometrium due to ↓ progesterone and ↓ estradiol

How is estrogen synthesized?

Cholesterol
   ↓ *cholesterol desmolase*
Pregnenolone
   ↓
   ↓
   ↓
Androstenedione
   ↓ *21-β-hydroxylase*
Testosterone
   ↓ *aromatase*
Estradiol

Name the actions of estrogen.

Maturation of fallopian tubes, uterus, cervix, and vagina

Puberty

♀ secondary sexual characteristics: growth of breasts

Development of granulosa cells

Maintenance of pregnancy: suppression of uterine response to contractile stimuli and prolactin secretion

Both positive and negative feedback on FSH and LH secretion

Up-regulation of LH, estrogen, and progesterone receptors

Name the actions of progesterone.

Maintenance of pregnancy: suppression of uterine response to contractile stimuli

Maintenance of luteal phase and uterine secretory activity

Negative feedback on FSH and LH

What factors regulate the menstrual. cycle, estrogen and progesterone secretion?

1. GnRH
2. FSH and LH
3. Estrogen (negative feedback)
4. Estrogen (positive feedback—ovulation)
5. Progesterone (negative feedback)

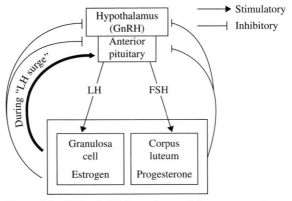

Figure 8.4 HPG axis. LH Surge is one of the rare examples of positive hormonal feedback.

PHYSIOLOGY OF PREGNANCY

How long after intercourse does fertilization occur?

Several hours; sperm uses a swimming motion to propel itself toward the fallopian tube and uterine and fallopian contraction during the female orgasm assists in drawing the sperm toward the waiting egg

What is the name of the fertilization product?

A zygote; the cellular union of the sperm and egg leads to genetic fusion, this fusion is called syngamy

How long after fertilization does implantation occur?

The blastocyst implants approximately 7 days after fertilization

What is happening to the zygote between fertilization and implantation?

Cell divisions; the zygote undergoes several divisions with a 70 to 100 cell product.

The other important event is the continued development of the uterine endometrium. It is in the secretory phase under the influence of the corpus luteum

Describe the blastocyst.

It is a collection of cells, the trophoblastic cells, that is arranged into a spherical shell with an inner cell mass that will ultimately develop into the embryo.

Describe the process of implantation.

The trophoblastic shell comes into close proximity of the endometrium
↓
Specific ligand mediated interactions leads to adhesion of the blastocyst
↓
The trophoblast differentiate rapidly dividing into two populations: cytotrophoblasts and syncytiotrophoblasts
↓
The syncytiotrophoblasts rapidly invade the endometrium leading to definitive implantation

What are cytotrophoblasts?

These are the inner blastocyst cells that invade the endometrium as chorionic villi after the syncytiotrophoblast has securely anchored the placental unit

What is the name of the structure that facilitates maternal-fetal exchange?

The placenta

What are the two primary functions of the placenta?

1. A transport epithelium allowing for maternal-fetal exchange of nutrients and metabolic waste products
2. An endocrine gland

How do oxygen and carbon dioxide get across the placenta?

Passive diffusion

How does glucose move across the placenta?

Facilitated diffusion

How do vitamins, amino acids, and other nutrients get across the placenta?

Secondary active transport

Name the main hormone producers in pregnancy and their associated products.

Corpus luteum:
1. hCG
2. Estradiol
3. Progesterone (conception to ~week 12)

Fetal adrenal gland:
   DHEA-S

Placenta:
1. Estriol
2. Progesterone (week 6 to delivery)
3. HPL

How is estriol synthesized in pregnancy?

DHEA-S (fetal adrenals)
$\downarrow$ *aromatase*
Estriol (placenta)

How does maternal blood volume change during pregnancy?

It increases to accommodate placental perfusion, to provide a buffer against blood loss during childbirth, and to ensure adequate maternal venous return.

By what degree does the blood volume change?

It increases by approximately 40% to 50%

What happens to the hematocrit?

Because the volume change is mediated by the renin-angiotensin system, it is primarily an increase in plasma volume. This leads to a dilutional anemia.

What happens to maternal coagulability?

Pregnancy is considered a hypercoagulable state. There is an increase in coagulation factors to protect the mother from hemorrhage during childbirth.

In pregnancy, what happens to the immune system?	Cellular immunity is suppressed as a way to protect the fetus from maternal immune assault
During pregnancy, what happens to respiration?	Yes, alveolar ventilation increases through an increase in tidal volume.
What happens to the GI tract during pregnancy?	Progesterone tends to relax smooth muscle to allow for added uterine relaxation, as a consequence, GI smooth muscle also relaxes, some leading to the common complaint of constipation.
What other changes might we anticipate in pregnancy?	Increase in GFR to help clear fetal wastes
	Nutritional demands increase so that the body can manage all of the above changes. Most notable are the increase in folate needs and the iron needs to help deal with fetal growth
How long does pregnancy last in humans?	40 weeks

How do the concentrations of the following hormones change during pregnancy?

Pituitary:	
TSH	$\leftrightarrow$
LH and FSH	Basal level
GH	$\leftrightarrow$
PRL	$\uparrow$ to term
ACTH	$\leftrightarrow$
Placenta and fetus:	
Estradiol	$\uparrow$ to term
Estriol	$\uparrow$ to term
Estrone	$\uparrow$ to term
Progesterone	$\uparrow$ to term
HPL	$\uparrow$ to term
Maternal adrenals and ovaries:	
Testosterone	$\uparrow\uparrow\uparrow$
DHEA	$\downarrow$
Cortisol	$\uparrow$

What factors influence lactation?	↑ of PRL through pregnancy accompanied by the ↓ of estrogens and progesterones after delivery
How is lactation maintained?	By breast-feeding, which ↑ PRL and oxytocin
How is ovulation suppressed during lactation?	PRL inhibits GnRH and, therefore, LH and FSH

CLINICAL VIGNETTES

A 42-year-old man undergoes prostate surgery for a suspicious nodule. He now comes to your office requesting help with erection complaining that he can't have successful intercourse with his wife. What is the likely diagnosis and what types of drugs can you offer him?

Erectile dysfunction, a common complication of prostate surgeries. A class of drugs called phosphodiesterase inhibitors influence the tonal control of vascular smooth muscle by increasing cyclic GMP levels leading to prolonged vasodilation and prolonged engorgement.

A newborn infant is being examined in your newborn nursery. A medical student notices that the infant has a small amount of breast tissue and has been lactating small amounts of breast milk. What is the most likely explanation?

The circulating hormones during pregnancy can affect fetal tissues in the same way they affect maternal tissues

A mother brings her 7-year-old daughter to your office because she is concerned about the development of coarse underarm and pubic hair. What is this condition called?

Precocious puberty. Described as pubertal changes before the age of 8 in girls or before the age of 9 in boys. Signifies endogenous sex steroid production. The condition is important to treat promptly. Untreated patients will grow quickly and their growth plates will fuse prematurely

A young mother comes in eight months after giving birth to a healthy baby girl. Her postpartum period has been uneventful, but she and her husband have been trying to conceive again and have been unable. You discover that she has been breastfeeding her new daughter and her menstrual cycle has not yet returned. What do you tell her?

The suckling reaction leads to secretion of prolactin and oxytocin in young mothers. These hormones inhibit the GnRH release in the usual monthly cycle and thereby inhibit LH and FSH release. Without these your patient is not ovulating and cannot conceive. If she wishes to conceive you should tell her that she should stop breastfeeding and that her cycle should return in 2 to 3 months.

A curious 22-year-old who is eight months pregnant consults you wondering why, although her breasts have gotten significantly larger since conception, she has not yet produced milk. What do you tell her?

During pregnancy the lactation apparatus is optimized for milk production, however, prolactin and oxytocin, two key hormones required for lactation are inhibited by the high estrogen concentrations of pregnancy.

A researcher has become very interested in the female reproductive system. He has decided to study the hormones involved in ovulation. During what day of the menses would the researcher have to study in order to investigate the day of ovulation?

14 days before menses

While undergoing a removal of a neurological tumor, a young woman suffers damage to her hypothalamus leading to loss of gonadotropin-releasing hormone (GnRH) secretion. What hormone(s) would be directly affected by this?

Luteinizing hormone (LH) and follicle stimulating hormone (FSH)

A woman has been studying her ovulation cycle by measuring her basal body temperature. She finds that after ovulation her temperature begins to rise slowly. What hormone is responsible for this effect? How?

Progesterone. It has an effect on the hypothalamic thermoregulatory center.

During the process of menses, the endometrium is sloughed off. What two hormones are responsible for the action?

Withdrawal of estradiol and progesterone

Suggested Readings

Costanzo LA. *Physiology*. 2nd ed. Philadelphia, PA: Saunders; 2002.

Cunningham G, Leveno KJ, Bloom SL, Hauth JC, Rouse D, Spong C. *Williams Obstetrics*. 23rd ed. New York, NY: McGraw-Hill; 2010.

Fauci A, Braunwald E, Kasper DL, et al. *Harrison's Principles of Internal Medicine*. 17th ed. New York, NY: McGraw-Hill; 2008.

Ganong WF. *Review of Medical Physiology*. 23rd ed. New York, NY: McGraw-Hill; 2009.

Guyton AC, Hall JE. *Textbook of Medical Physiology*. 11th ed. Philadelphia, PA: Elsevier Saunders; 2005.

Kibble JD, Halsey CR. *Medical Physiology: The Big Picture*. New York, NY: McGraw-Hill; 2009.

Levitsky MG. *Pulmonary Physiology*. 7th ed. New York, NY: McGraw-Hill; 2007.

Mason RJ, Murray JF, Broaddus VC, Nadel JA. *Murray and Nadel's Textbook of Respiratory Medicine*. 4th ed. Philadelphia, PA: Elsevier Saunders; 2005.

Robbins SL, Cotran RS, Kumar V. *Robbins Pathologic Basis of Disease*. 6th ed. Philadelphia, PA: Saunders; 1999:1121-1168.

Silverthorn DU. *Human Physiology*. 3rd ed. San Francisco, CA: Pearson Education, Inc; 2004.

Index

Page numbers followed by *f* indicate figures; *t* tables.